In Great Shape

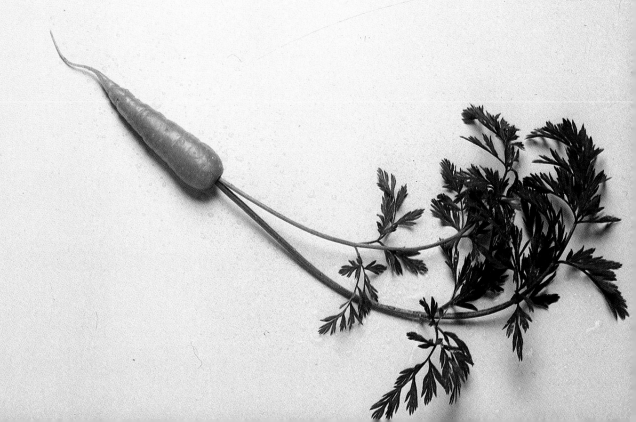

In Great Shape

A guide to diet and exercise

Arline Usden

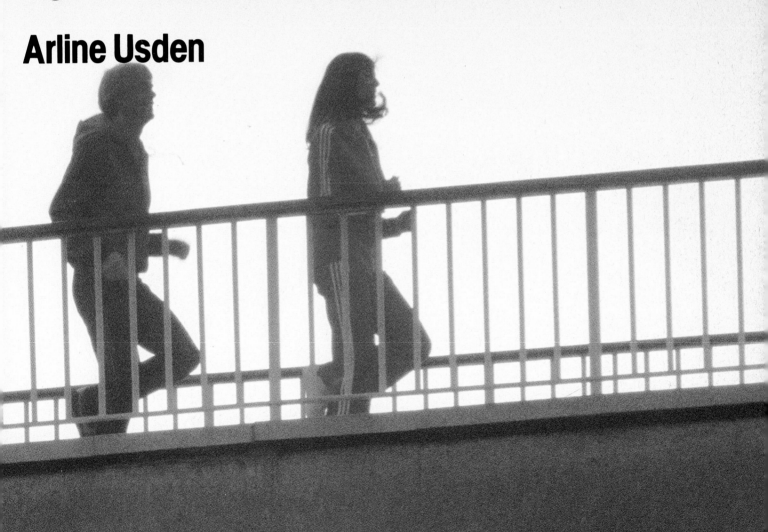

Artus

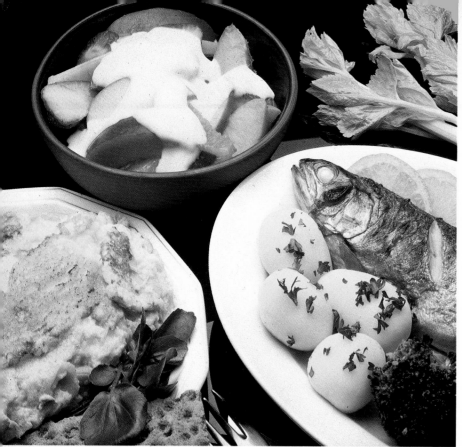

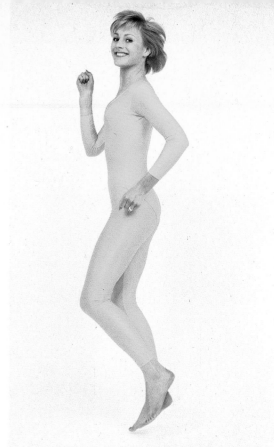

First published in 1981
Second Impression
August 1981
Third Impression
October 1981
Fourth Impression May
1982
by Artus Publishing
Company Ltd
91 Clapham High Street
London SW4 7TA

Design and art direction
by Kieran Stevens
Photography by Chris
Holland and Paul Kemp

Filmset by Keyspools Ltd,
Golborne, Lancs
Colour separations by
Newsele Litho Ltd
Printed in Hong Kong by
Mandarin Publishers Ltd

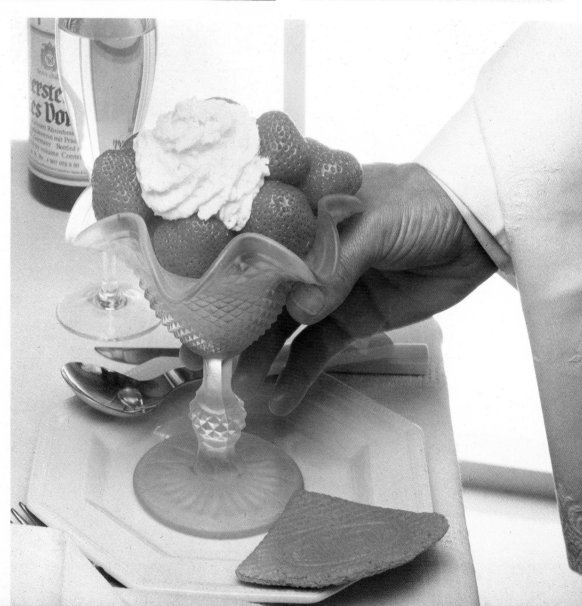

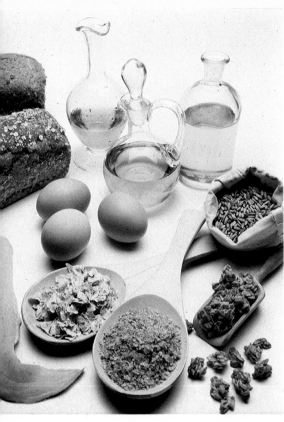

Contents

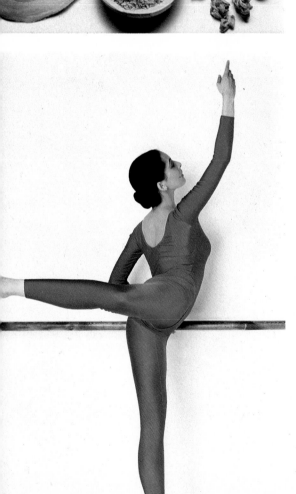

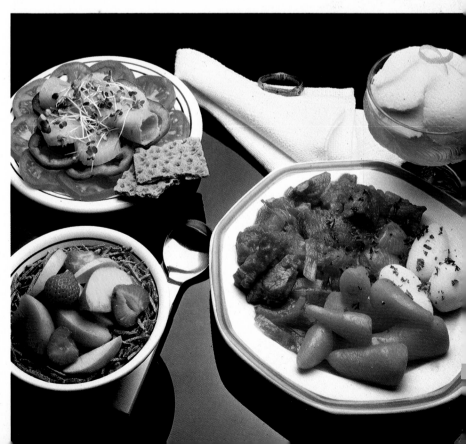

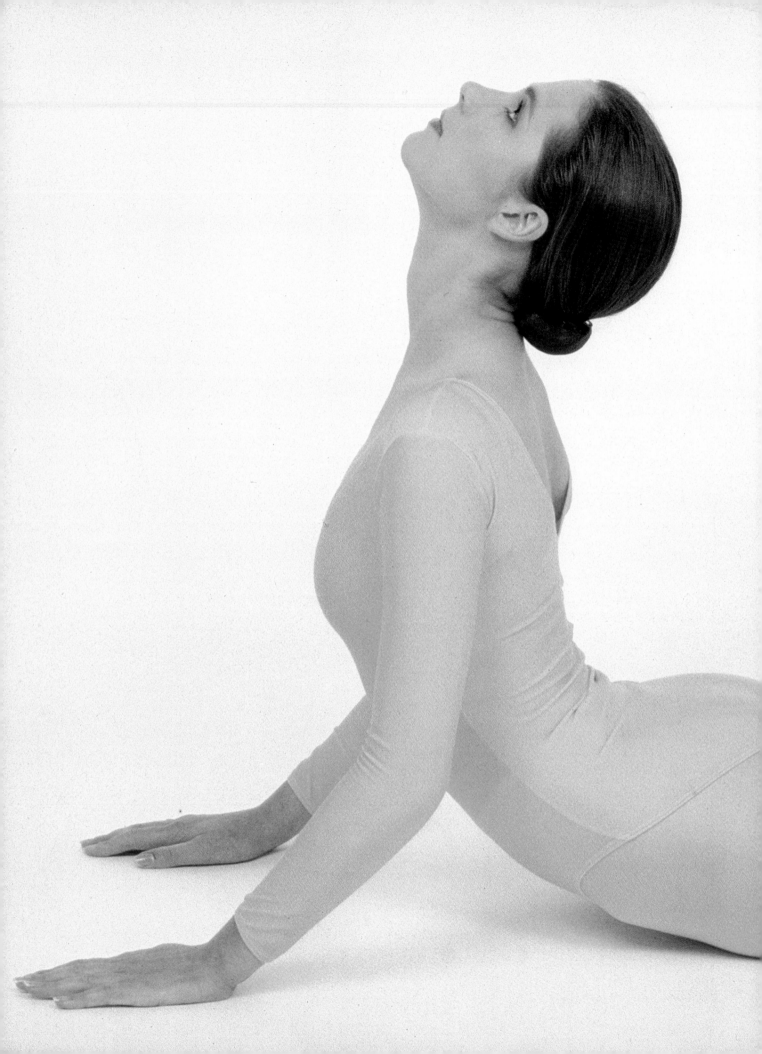

Introduction

How do you shape up to life? Are you slim, supple, full of energy and fit for anything? Or are you rather fat and unfit? If you are, you're by no means alone because about half the population seems to weigh more than is good for them and the figures of people trying to slim do not appear to change either physically or statistically! A weighty problem indeed when you consider that being overweight not only takes away some of the enjoyment of life, but also actually shortens it by contributing to ill health and disease.

Excess pounds, however, are only half the health and beauty story, because without the right balance of foods and without exercise you can never reach your full fitness potential. Today, doctors know that to reduce weight you should not only reduce your intake of calories, but also eat less fat, less sugar and salt, more fibre, fresh vegetables and fruit; and that you should exercise not just for a beautifully trim and toned-up body and strength, but also for your heart and lungs.

If fat means unfit, it certainly doesn't seem bad for business, as you can see from all the slimming notions and gadgets aimed at staking up your willpower. During my years as a Beauty Editor, I must have tried or had tested just about every new health and slimming idea, from jumping up and down in plastic 'slimming pants' to having my bulges 'ironed' out with electric massagers. I can assure you that most of them do not work. You cannot lose weight by rubbing creams into your skin, by taking hot bubble baths, by wrapping up in warm wax or by eating half a grapefruit before every meal. Taking a substitute meal diet-biscuit or milkshake is no way to retrain yourself into better balanced eating habits, I'm afraid, and there is (as yet) no magic solution or pill that can instantly change you from a wobbly oversized 18 into a pretty little size 8, without *you* making the effort.

But diets do not have to have overtones of martyrdom and self-denial, and exercise can be fun and relaxing both to mind and body. I believe any woman can become slimmer, fitter and more energetic, whatever her age, but I also know that the biggest problem of all is getting started! I hope this book will give you the incentive to plough through the Slimming Jungle and *succeed*.

Weighing it Up

Your Shape

The way you look has a lot to do with your ancestors, your nutrition and your environment. Our genetic inheritance is far from simple, but like still produces like, and if you come from a long line of small, fairly tubby people, you are probably not going to resemble a tall, slender model. Nutrition also affects your average height. In Britain, for example, the post-war generation was nearly two inches taller than the generation born before 1930 because of a better, more balanced diet. Environment, the third factor, is particularly important in your early years: children brought up in love and security will grow more than those on a similar diet but with fewer emotional advantages.

Body types fall into three basic categories. *The endomorph* has a rounded shape (including the head), a heavy build and a lot of fat. Even if not obese, the endomorph will always be softly rounded, and is supposed to be easy-going and relaxed.

The ectomorph is sharp and thin, with spindly legs and arms, narrow shoulders and hips, not much muscle or fat. Ectomorphs are said to be sensitive and tense.

The mesomorph is more athletic, with a lot of bone and muscle but not much fat. This type has a large head, broad shoulders and relatively narrow hips, and tends to be aggressive and competitive.

Most of us, of course, are a combination of the three types, with a slant towards one

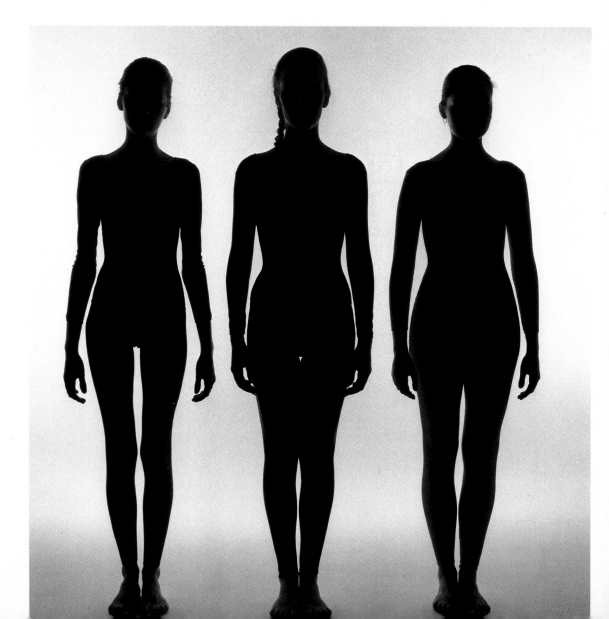

Left to right, an ectomorph, a mesomorph and an endomorph. Most people are a combination of the three body types.

8

particular shape. Your body type stays with you all your life, and although you can change the amount of fat under your skin and your general all-over plumpness or leanness, you will never alter your basic shape. A well-balanced diet combined with exercise can, however, improve your muscle-tone, and make the very best of what nature has given you.

Your Weight

It's easy to fool yourself into thinking that you are not overweight. 'Heavy bones', 'nicely covered', 'generous proportions' are all phrases that we use to disguise the fact of our fatness. But in order to lose weight and, having lost it, maintain your ideal level, you must learn to assess yourself honestly. So how can you tell whether you're deceiving yourself?

Look at yourself
Stand naked in front of a full-length mirror and look at yourself from the front, back and sides. Take the shades from your eyes and face the truth of the situation. Does your flesh wobble and seem dimpled? Can you see the bulges? Are your thighs very thick? Does your stomach stick out?

Try the pinch test
Although this is most accurate when done by doctors or slimming experts using skinfold calipers, it's still a good indication of excess weight, and easy to do. Pinch a fold of skin at the back of your upper arm (half way between your elbow and shoulder), an inch above your waist (in the front), and on the side of your leg where the hip meets the thigh. If the thickness of the pinched skin in any of these places is more than one inch, you are overweight. Bear in mind that the average *healthy* woman has 22 per cent body weight as fat; the average woman has more like 32 per cent body fat. If you can pinch the inch, roughly 40 pounds of your body weight is fat. That doesn't mean that you have to lose all of it, because the subcutaneous fat under your skin is what pads out your body and gives you womanly curves. But it does mean you have some weight to lose.

Weigh yourself regularly
Weight tables are a good but not infallible guide. The target table on this page is based on several expert sources and is more realistic than many of the tables produced by insurance companies, which usually seem to give very generous weight allowances. Try to weigh yourself about once a week at the same time of day, and preferably without clothes. Make sure your scales are standing on a smooth, flat surface – carpets can make weighing machines inaccurate and cause fluctuations.

Be realistic
Have you ever taken a smaller size in clothes? How do you look in a swimsuit? Could you wear a bikini? Have any of your clothes become too tight for you? Remember that when you can't do up the zip of your jeans one day, it does not necessarily mean that your trousers have shrunk.

Fat Times of your Life

Being overweight seems to run in families, probably because everyone is eating the same kind of diet and, genetically, they are not good 'burners' of energy. Today, you won't find the chubbiest baby winning the Beautiful Baby competition because doctors know that it is wrong to encourage fatness in children. An overweight baby often becomes an obese adult; and the first 12 months are crucial.
Babies Bottle-fed babies may run a greater risk of becoming too fat than breast-fed babies, because the mother may measure out food inaccurately and add cereals too early.
Children Although overeating, combined with less utilization of energy, leads to fatness, fat children do not necessarily overeat. Often

TARGET WEIGHT TABLE			
HEIGHT	SMALL FRAME	MEDIUM FRAME	LARGE FRAME
ft in	st lb (lbs)	st lb (lbs)	st lb (lbs)
4 8	6 8 (92)	6 13 (97)	7 8 (106)
4 9	6 10 (94)	7 1 (99)	7 11 (109)
4 10	7 0 (98)	7 7 (105)	8 1 (113)
4 11	7 3 (101)	7 11 (109)	8 4 (116)
5 0	7 6 (104)	8 0 (112)	8 7 (119)
5 1	7 9 (107)	8 2 (114)	8 10 (122)
5 2	7 12 (110)	8 5 (117)	8 13 (125)
5 3	8 1 (113)	8 8 (120)	9 2 (128)
5 4	8 5 (117)	8 12 (124)	9 6 (132)
5 5	8 7 (119)	9 1 (127)	9 10 (136)
5 6	8 11 (123)	9 5 (131)	10 0 (140)
5 7	9 1 (127)	9 9 (135)	10 3 (143)
5 8	9 4 (130)	9 13 (139)	10 7 (147)
5 9	9 8 (134)	10 3 (143)	10 11 (151)
5 10	9 11 (137)	10 6 (146)	11 0 (154)
5 11	10 1 (141)	10 10 (150)	11 5 (159)
6 0	10 5 (145)	10 13 (153)	11 10 (164)

This table is a general guide for women. Determine your type of frame by measuring your wrist. If it is 140 mm (5½ in) or less, you have a small frame; 140–160 mm (5½–6½ in), a medium frame; more than 160 mm (6½ in), a large frame. The weights given are without clothes, and height should be measured without shoes.

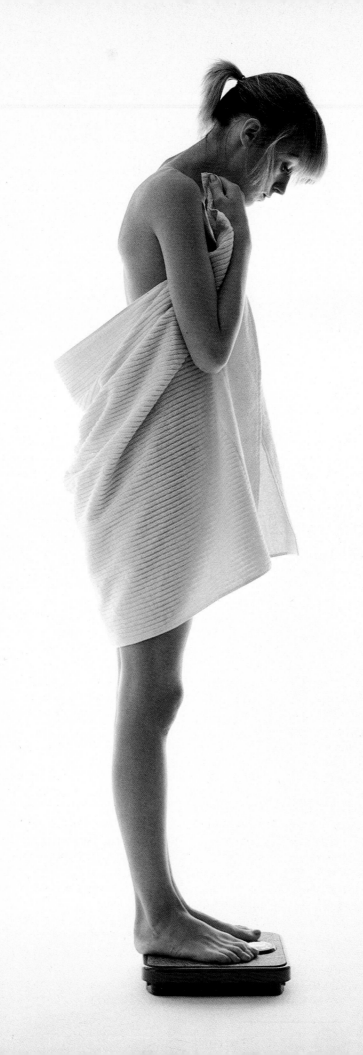

they simply use less energy than slimmer children because their movements are slower and they are less active. Fat children are not as popular at school as thinner, more athletic children; they are usually not good at games and feel embarrassed stripping down to sports clothes: all reasons to encourage a sensible eating pattern.

Teenagers   Hormonal changes at adolescence mean that girls put on fat and change shape in a pattern which isn't pleasing to them. Being teased is wounding, emotionally. But childhood fatness can also leave scars physically, when stretched skin leaves stretch marks even when the fatness has gone. It's an unwise mother who says 'Eat up and ignore it – it's only puppy fat.' A relaxed but sensible attitude towards family eating can help to win the battle of the bulges before it gets out of control.

Marriage   Cooking for a husband, having a settled life, trying to produce interesting meals, giving dinner parties, shopping, more time to nibble . . . all these can lead to putting on weight. For some women, alas, going to the altar satisfies an ambition, and standards drop afterwards because they've lost their incentive to food discipline.

Pregnancy   Having a baby is naturally one of the fattest times in a woman's life. 'Eating for two', you may say, taking the opportunity to eat whatever you like, whenever you like. But the maximum amount of weight you should put on is about 24 pounds. Doctors encourage a sensible attitude to diet, because too much weight can lead to a risk of complications.

Motherhood   A mother of young children seems to be surrounded by food all day long. Eating up left-overs is very tempting, and the opportunities to nibble are endless. See page 36 for ways to help your willpower.

Getting older   Generally, the older we become, the less active we are, and older people need fewer calories from food. You should make a positive effort to get more exercise or, if that's not possible, reduce the amount you eat.

There are also factors other than age which can affect your weight at certain times.

The pill   The hormones in birth control pills could encourage the body to retain more liquid and to lay down more stores of fat. Discuss any tendency to put on weight with your doctor, who may prescribe a different kind of pill.

Your state of mind   The reason for a sudden spurt of weight may be a psychological one. You might find that when you feel more relaxed you increase your appetite. Or you could be the kind of person who overeats when depressed, as compensation; if being overweight depresses you, you could find yourself caught in a vicious circle that's hard to break.

Some women find that being in love takes away their appetite. They have other things in mind than food! An unhappy love affair, however, may lead to self-indulgence.

Giving up smoking   The oral satisfaction of a cigarette could be hard to give up and as smoking can dull your appetite, you may well find you have a healthier appetite when you quit. But do *not* be put off and certainly do not use any weight-gain as an excuse to carry on smoking. Lots of people give up and don't put on weight. If you need something in your mouth chew one of the slimmers' chewing gums, without sugar, or eat a carrot.

Why You Should Slim

Doctors consider you to be obese if you are more than 15 per cent heavier than your ideal weight for your height and build. Obesity affects about one in five people; many more are simply a little overweight. Most people go on diets purely for cosmetic reasons: they want to look better, feel more attractive, be able to wear the latest fashions. There are, however, very strong medical reasons for taking off that excess weight.

● The more overweight you are, the higher your chances of getting high blood pressure, diabetes, gallstones, bronchitis, arthritis, varicose veins, and heart attacks. Very obese people may also have a high level of cholesterol in the bloodstream, which may be closely linked with heart disease.

● Fat people are more prone to accidents. They find it difficult to move quickly or easily.

● Life insurance companies regularly load the policies of fat people because statistics show that anyone who is 20 per cent more than ideal weight has a greater chance of dying earlier than a person of the same age but normal weight.

● Surgeons will find it more difficult to operate on you if you are obese.

● Your bones and joints will take greater strain when you are very obese, which leads to other problems.

● Psychologically, being overweight leads to feelings of inadequacy and depression; it can ruin your love-life, destroy self-confidence and self-esteem. The image of the fat, jolly, easy-going person is not necessarily true. It could be a front, put up in self-defence.

● Fatness stops you being fit. You cannot exercise easily, will find it difficult to run. The fatter you are, the more difficult it is to move, which means your heart does not get the chance to be properly exercised, and you become breathless and strained with any effort.

Opposite: Weigh yourself regularly, without any clothes on. Keeping the scales on a bare floor rather than a carpet or rug helps to ensure accuracy of measurement.

The Energy Balance

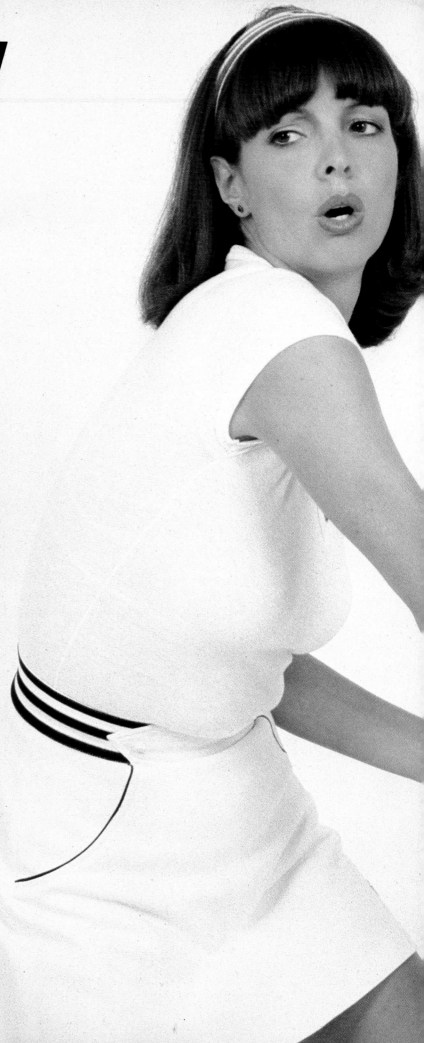

Just as a car is fuelled with petrol to produce energy, so the human body is fuelled with food, which is composed of carbohydrates, proteins and fats, our three main nutrients. These foods are converted into energy and their energy value in units of heat is calculated in calories (or joules when we go metric).

Every minute of our lives, sleeping or working, we burn up energy – more or less depending on the degree of effort and our metabolism. Some people are 'fast-burners', using up more energy than they consume, and stay slim no matter how much they eat. Others are 'sleepers', using up fewer calories than they take in, and get fat. What turns you into a fast burner or a sleeper? Scientists now have a theory that it's all to do with the special kind of brown adipose fat found at the base of the neck between the shoulder blades.

It is this special fat which helps to burn up all the surplus energy we consume as food. Fat people, it appears, do not have enough brown fat – and that's one of the reasons why some lucky people can scoff themselves silly on all kinds of fattening foods without putting on an inch, while less fortunate people put on weight after eating only an extra piece of bread. Scientists are investigating the means of stimulating the growth of this amazing brown fat and when they succeed – if they succeed – it could be the end of the obesity problem. Until that happens, I'm afraid diet-and-exercise is the only way to get rid of surplus weight.

The key to maintaining your ideal body weight, as an adult, is to balance the calories you take in against those you expend, rather like a bank account. When you regularly take in more energy than you need to use, your body converts the energy into fat and stores it in fat cells. These lie underneath your skin, and in addition to fat they contain water and other substances. Their number doesn't change, but they shrink or expand according to the amount of fat they contain. Obesity is when your body stock-piles far too much of this fat. When you regularly take in fewer calories than you burn, you lose weight as your body calls on its fat storage for energy.

Calorie Requirements

Your own daily energy requirement depends on your body size, sex, age, and the degree of physical activity you undertake. Women tend to need less energy than men, although needs are increased during pregnancy and breast-feeding. Manual workers use more calories than those who sit at desks all day. Older people tend to need fewer calories than younger ones. The amount of calories you use up in physical activity depends on your weight and how strenuously you work or play. A heavy man will burn up more calories playing a game of tennis than a lighter woman because he is heavier, not necessarily because he runs about more. Cycling up hills and running instead of walking will use up more calories than a gentle stroll or bike ride.

The table on this page is a general guide to your daily maximum calorie requirement once you have reached your ideal weight. If you want to do your own calculation, multiply your ideal weight (in pounds) by 12 if you live a sedentary, non-active kind of life; by 15 if you are moderately active; and by 18 if you are very active. You may find that you can afford to eat a little more and stay the same; or that you have to reduce your calorie intake to maintain weight. It all depends on whether you are a fast fat burner or a slow burner.

We expend calories in energy even while we are sleeping, sustaining the basic functions of life such as breathing and blood circulation, and we move around quite a lot in our sleep. A woman of 5 feet 4 inches weighing 131 pounds would use up about 520 calories during a night's sleep – nearly equivalent to two hours' horseriding or six hours' ironing. It's surprising, though, how much activity is required to work off that little snack which we knew we shouldn't have but didn't really think would matter. In terms of your energy balance, a small packet of peanuts can equal an hour of badminton, a small portion of chips an hour of bowling.

MAXIMUM DAILY CALORIE REQUIREMENTS

AGE	FEMALE
12–15	2300
15–18	2300
18–35	
Sedentary	2200
Quite active	2350
Very active	2500
35–60	
Sedentary	2200
Quite active	2350
Very active	2500
60–75	
Sedentary	2050
Quite active	2250
Very active	2350
Over 75	1900

CALORIE EXPENDITURE IN MINUTES

	Calories	Cycling 24 km (15 m) per hour	Gardening	Golf	Running 12 km (7.5 m) per hour	Swimming 41 metres (45 yards) per minute	Tennis	Walking 4 km (2.5 m) per hour	Housework
225 ml (8 fl oz) cola drink	88	9	18	22	8	9	13	18	35
280 ml (½ pint) dry cider	100	10	20	25	9	10	14	20	40
25 g (1 oz) toffees	123	12	25	31	11	12	18	25	49
25 g (1 oz) crisps	152	14	30	38	14	15	22	30	61
25 g (1 oz) peanuts	163	16	33	41	15	16	23	33	65
55 g (2 oz) Cheddar cheese	232	22	46	58	21	23	33	46	93
1 croissant	270	26	54	67	25	27	39	54	108
1 chocolate milkshake	365	35	73	91	33	33	52	73	146

Above right: This table is a general guide to daily requirements for women. Those who are pregnant and reasonably active need about 2400 calories; when breast-feeding after birth, this rises to about 2700.

Above: This table shows how long you would have to spend at each of nine activities to use up the average calorie intake of ten fairly fattening snacks.

Eating for Health

The food you eat provides materials for three main purposes. For growth and repair of body tissues, meals must include protein, minerals and vitamins. For protection and maintenance of good health, meals must include vitamins, minerals and water. For energy and warmth, meals must include carbohydrates and fats. Sometimes, the body uses protein as a fuel if no other source is available.

The Nutrients

Proteins, carbohydrates and fats are called major nutrients because we need them in relatively large amounts.

Protein
Besides water, protein is the most abundant substance in the body cells. It is made up of carbon, hydrogen and nitrogen and occasionally sulphur and phosphorus. It helps to build and repair the body and accounts for the tough, fibrous nature of hair, nails, ligaments and muscles. It forms part of the haemoglobin (red blood cells), the digestive enzymes and insulin, and is made up of about 22 amino acids (10 of these cannot be made by the body). The digestive enzymes break down the protein we eat into constituent amino acids and the body uses these to manufacture its own protein.

If we take in more protein than we need for body building, the extra supply may be burned up as energy or converted into body fat. Actually, most of us today in the affluent West eat far more protein than we need – about 50g ($1\frac{3}{4}$ oz) a day would be enough, for health.

Because the composition of animal tissue is most similar to our own, meat, milk, eggs, cheese, poultry and fish contain a more correct balance of amino acids than the plant proteins such as peas, beans, nuts, cereals and cereal products. Most plant sources are usually low in one essential amino acid: vegetarians should be careful to eat a wide variety of plants which will complement one another and increase the total value of the protein intake.

Called the building blocks of the body, protein makes up about 12 per cent of our weight.

Carbohydrates
Much cheaper to obtain than protein, carbohydrates provide much of the world's population with about 70 per cent of its energy, although this figure is much lower (about 40 per cent) in Western countries. Obtained from sugar and starches, they are chemical compounds of carbon, hydrogen and oxygen.

Starch forms the larger proportion of the carbohydrates we eat in our food. It must be broken down by the body into sugars before it can be used for energy. Carbohydrates begin in plants with the action of sunlight on plant leaves (photosynthesis) which produces plant sap in the form of simple sugars. This is later converted into starch and forms the plant's own store of fuel. The starch may be further condensed into cellulose, which forms the fibrous parts of plants and trees. Human digestive enzymes are unable to break down the complex structure of cellulose and it is therefore not available to us as direct energy, although it is useful in the diet – and is now increasingly respected – as a source of necessary roughage. We consume most of our starch in breads, cereals, potatoes, flour, pasta and rice.

Sugar is another source of energy. In the body, more complex sugars and starch are broken down into glucose, and this is the form in which fuel is transported round the organs. Fructose is the sweetest type of sugar known and occurs naturally in plant juices and honey. Sucrose is the substance we normally refer to as sugar. It occurs naturally in sugar beet and sugar cane and is the fuel store of these plants. Lactose or milk sugar occurs naturally in animal and human milk and is used in margarine and butter manufacture. Maltose is formed naturally from starch during the germination of grain and in the production of malt liquors. Today, we eat about five times more sugar than 100 years ago, and as much in two weeks as people 200 years ago ate in one year. It doesn't really matter what kind it is. White or brown, maple syrup or molasses, it is still sugar. All sugar is empty calories because it supplies nothing but energy to the diet. It should be part of your day's intake in moderation only, never in excess. The benefits of honey and health-food syrups are just part of the myths of the food world; there's nothing in them that you cannot obtain normally and easily elsewhere in your diet. You may like the taste, but the effect on the body and your teeth is the same as pure sucrose – and dentists now say that

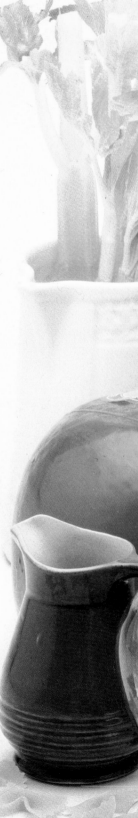

sugar is the *only* reason for tooth decay. The trouble with sweetstuff is that it's addictive. You get a quick, short burst of energy and then you feel flat. On a slimming diet you should replace sugar by low or non-calorie synthetic sweeteners or, better by far, retrain your palate and cut down on sweet things altogether. Since much of our sugar consumption is through foods high in fat (ice cream, cakes, biscuits), this will be even more beneficial to your health.

Fats

Made up of carbon, hydrogen and oxygen, fats provide a concentrated source of energy for the body since their energy value is twice that of proteins and carbohydrates. This makes them a high-calorie food. In addition to providing energy, fats also assist the transport of fat-soluble vitamins around the body. They prevent the onset of hunger after a meal as they are slow to digest, and they make linoleic acid, which is necessary for healthy skin.

Fats are composed of fatty acids and glycerol. Chemically, each fatty acid is made up of chains of carbon atoms which have hydrogen atoms attached to them. When each carbon atom has the maximum possible number of hydrogen atoms attached, it is known as saturated fat. Different patterns of carbon/hydrogen atoms produce: mono-unsaturated and polyunsaturated fats.

Around 40 per cent of the calories in our diet are supplied by fats. Recent reports from medical bodies regard this as too high, recommending that it should be reduced to no more than 35 per cent. And some experts now believe that it is particularly helpful to reduce levels of *saturated* fats in the diet, because they are one of the known risk factors said to contribute to the rise of high blood cholesterol (see below), and coronary heart disease.

In the diet, fats are divided into visible ones, like butter and lard, and invisible ones – present in foods such as meat and fatty fish, eggs, cakes, biscuits and pastry. Saturated fats include animal fats (lard, suet, dripping), butter, hard cheeses and hard margarine, all of which remain solid at room temperature, and cream, full fat milk and coconut oil. Olive oil and ground-nut oil are mono-unsaturated fats. Polyunsaturated fats are so soft that they will not solidify even in the fridge, and include sunflower oil, corn oil, safflower oil, cotton-seed oil, soyabean oil and soft margarines marked high in polyunsaturates. Most nuts (not coconuts or cashews) are also polyun-saturated. The saturated *vs* unsaturated fats controversy is likely to continue; if in doubt, simply reduce the intake of *total* fats in your diet.

Cholesterol is a fat-like substance which is produced naturally in the bodies of all animals, including man. Although essential, we produce enough for our own purposes and, strictly speaking, don't need to eat any to stay healthy.

A high level of cholesterol in the blood stream encourages the build-up of deposits of fat on the inside walls of the arteries, which makes the channels of the arteries narrower and interferes with the blood supply to the heart. This can sometimes lead to a heart attack. Consistently high amounts of cholesterol in food *may* increase the level of cholesterol in the blood stream, but this level is

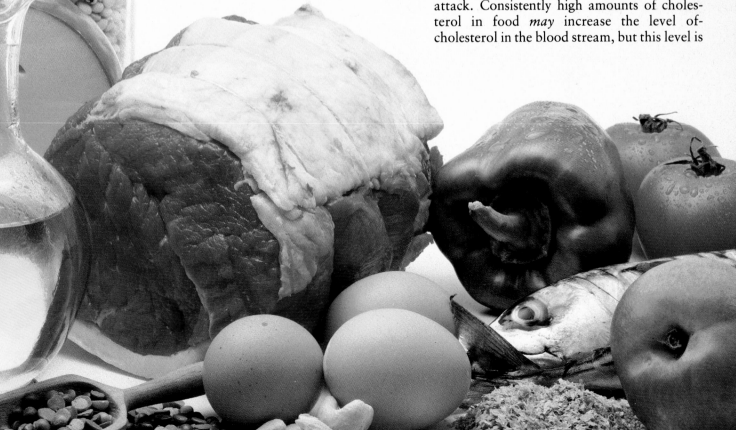

affected more by the type of fat we eat. Foods which contain a lot of hard, saturated fat can raise the blood cholesterol level. Soft or polyunsaturated fats can help to lower the amount of cholesterol in the blood. Egg yolks are a rich source of cholesterol; liver, kidneys, shellfish, butter and cream also contain a lot.

Fibre

Fibre, or roughage, absorbs many times its own weight in water and thus provides bulk in the bowel which exercises the muscles of the large intestine, making bowel action more regular and easier. The importance of fibre in our diet has been increasingly confirmed by doctors in recent years, and lack of it is now considered to contribute to several diseases and ailments, notably constipation but also from diverticular disease (when the bowel becomes obstructed), haemorrhoids and cancer of the rectum to varicose veins and heart disease. Because of this, coarse, unrefined bread and potatoes have been rescued from their Cinderella status and are recommended by nutritionists as part of a good balanced calorie-controlled diet.

Good sources of fibre include wholemeal bread, bran breakfast cereals, pulses such as beans, peas and lentils, potatoes, swedes, parsnips, carrots, turnips and bananas. Remember that brown bread isn't necessarily wholemeal, which contains all the bran and fibre of the cereals. Some brown breads are made from partly refined flour, with about half the bran removed – though they still have more fibre than white bread.

Vitamins and Minerals

Are you getting your fair share of vitamins and minerals? It's a question we probably ask ourselves quite often because so much is written and talked about these invisible, potent and seemingly magical elements in our food. However, a good deal of this is myth, hearsay and exaggeration, so it's as well to examine the claims more closely before you reach for that box of multi-vitamin pills.

Vitamins are essential organic substances which are involved in body metabolism. We need them in small amounts; deficiency of any one vitamin may result in disease. Minerals are inorganic substances, several of which are essential – again in small amounts – to our diet. Iron, for instance, helps to form our red blood cells; calcium is necessary for strong bones and teeth. Since much of the talk about vitamins and minerals concerns deficiencies, it's important to remember that there can be a danger of over-compensation; vitamins A and D and some minerals can be harmful if taken in large quantities.

If you eat a well-balanced diet which includes fresh foods, you are probably not suffering from any deficiencies. There are, however, factors other than diet which can influence this:

● Aspirin is said to lead to iron deficiency in people who take it regularly, caused by small but repeated losses of blood in the bowel through irritation of the lining of the stomach. Aspirin may also lead to some reduction in the level of vitamin C in the blood, as will antibiotics such as tetracyclines.

● Smoking may be associated with lower blood plasma levels of vitamin C and vitamin B_{12}.

● Oral contraceptives, depending on the pill used, may sometimes increase blood cholesterol and cause pyridoxine (vitamin B_6) deficiency, resulting in depression.

● If you take laxatives too regularly you could lose excessive amounts of potassium.

● Eating a limited diet high in refined carbohydrates has been shown to lead to a deficiency in vitamin B_1.

● If you are an alcoholic, you may be short of the B vitamins and folic acid.

● If you eat a lot of carbohydrates and drink a great deal of alcohol too, you will probably need more vitamin B_1 to help metabolize food energy.

Some vitamins, such as B and C, are water-soluble and sensitive to heat. In order to retain the vitamin content of vegetables, either steam them or boil them for just a short time in very little water. More vitamins are probably lost through careless home cooking than through modern processing methods – which retain far more vitamins in food than some food faddists would care to admit.

There is still a good deal of controversy about whether high vitamin C supplements help prevent the common cold, or mitigate the symptoms. Some people say that utilization of vitamin C is abnormal during bouts of a cold, hay fever and asthma, and that an extra dose is beneficial. Others maintain that taking massive doses of vitamins is based on the assumption that if a small amount is good for you, then a larger amount must be even better. But a large dose of one vitamin could produce side effects – perhaps blocking the body's ability to use another. And with a water-soluble vitamin, excess is simply excreted through the kidneys. The answer? Keep taking your vitamin C, preferably in the form of natural foods, but leave the mega-dose supplements until benefits are proven more conclusively. In winter, make sure you have plenty of fruit and vegetables, or natural fruit juice.

Vitamin and source	Function	Vitamin and source	Function

Vitamin A (retinol)
Oily fish such as sardines and herrings; butter, margarine, liver, kidneys, carrots, green vegetables such as spinach and watercress, tomatoes. The body can store a certain amount. Fat-soluble.

Necessary for growth, function of eyes, health of the skin.

Vitamin A

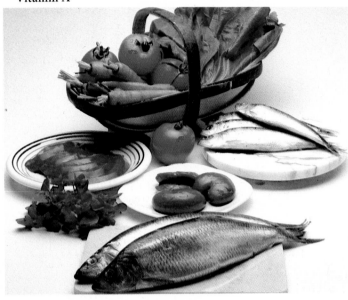

Vitamin B includes a complex of vitamins.

Vitamin B_1 (thiamin)
Wholemeal 'bread and cereals containing wheatgerm, liver, kidneys, heart, fish roe, eggs, yeast, soya flour, dried peas, raw beans, lean pork, lentils. Water-soluble, so can be destroyed in cooking.

Helps the nervous system to function. Controls release of energy from carbohydrate foods. Deficiency causes the nervous complaint called beri-beri.

Vitamin B_2 (riboflavin)
Cheese, eggs, herring, lentils, liver, kidneys, milk, vegetables. Resistant to heat but sunlight destroys it – keep milk from standing in the sun too long.

For energy, health of mouth, tongue, lips, skin.

Vitamin B_4 (niacin)
Brewers' yeast, liver, meat, bread, mushrooms, vegetables. One of most stable vitamins, hardly affected by cooking, freezing, canning or drying.

Crucial for energy, skin health. Deficiency produces pellagra, a disease where the skin turns dark and scaly.

Pantothenic acid
Liver, kidney, egg yolk, vegetables. Present in almost all types of food. Up to 50 per cent can be destroyed by cooking and canning, but not by freezing.

Essential for nervous system, and in the burning up of fat for energy.

Vitamin B_6 (pyridoxine)
Brewers' yeast, wholegrain cereals and bread, liver, milk, eggs, leafy vegetables. About 35 per cent is destroyed by cooking and canning.

Helps many body functions, from cell health to nerves. Mega-doses have been used successfully at clinics in the treatment of severe pre-menstrual tension.

Folic acid
Liver, kidneys, fresh green vegetables, nuts, oysters. Heat-sensitive; overcooking destroys a lot of it.

Important for red blood cells. Deficiency causes anaemia.

Vitamin B_{12}
Liver, kidneys, meat, dairy products such as milk, cheese. Can be stored in the liver. Raw egg white destroys it but this is unlikely in normal diet.

For production of red blood cells. Deficiency, although rare, can lead to anaemia.

Biotin
Yeast, kidneys, liver, egg yolk. Our own body produces it naturally, too.

For skin and hair particularly.

Vitamin B

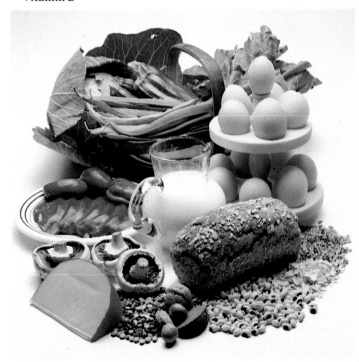

Vitamin C (ascorbic acid)
Vegetables of every kind – potatoes, cabbage and brussels sprouts are all good sources – fruit, especially citrus fruit and blackcurrants. Very sensitive to heat, easily destroyed by cooking, canning. You need some every day because the body does not store the vitamin. You may need more if you smoke.

Helps healing and resistance to infection; formation of healthy skin; promotes absorption of iron. Controls ability of body cells to produce collagen, the substance that binds cells together.

Vitamin and source	Function	Mineral and source	Function

Vitamin D (calciferol)
Margarine, butter, fatty fish liver. The vitamin is also produced in the body when there is exposure to sunlight. Can be stored in the body.

Aids absorption of calcium, needed for bone formation and teeth. Deficiency can lead to rickets in children.

Calcium
Milk, cheese, hard water (can sometimes supply up to half daily intake), fish such as sardines where bones are eaten, bread.

Necessary for the bones, teeth. Inadequate diet can cause problems in growth for the very young and in decay the very old.

Vitamin D

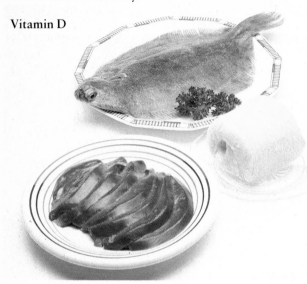

Calcium

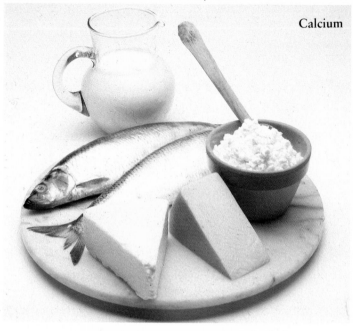

Vitamin E (tocopherol)
In many foods, particularly wholemeal bread and cereals, vegetable oils, eggs, fish. Much can be destroyed by deep frying.

A tissue protector, necessary for blood cells, maintenance of membranes.

Cobalt
A trace element, forms part of the Vitamin B_{12} molecule. Green vegetables, fruit, meat, cereals.

Control of metabolism, red blood cells, spinal cord.

Chromium
Seafood, wholegrain cereals, green vegetables, chicken, fruit, bran. A trace element.

Metabolism of sugars.

Vitamin K

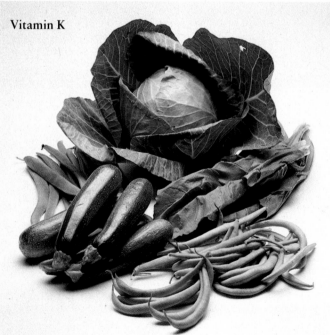

Chromium

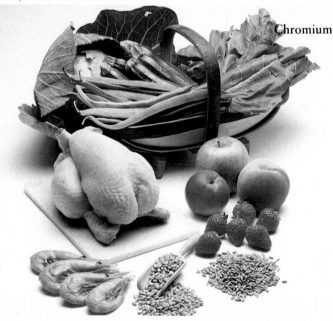

Vitamin K
Green leafy plants in particular. We make much of our own with the aid of natural bacteria in the intestine. Fat-soluble, it passes into blood-stream from intestine.

Aids clotting of blood.

Copper
Liver, dried fruit, searood, wholegrain cereals, almonds.

In traces, helps blood formation, hair pigment.

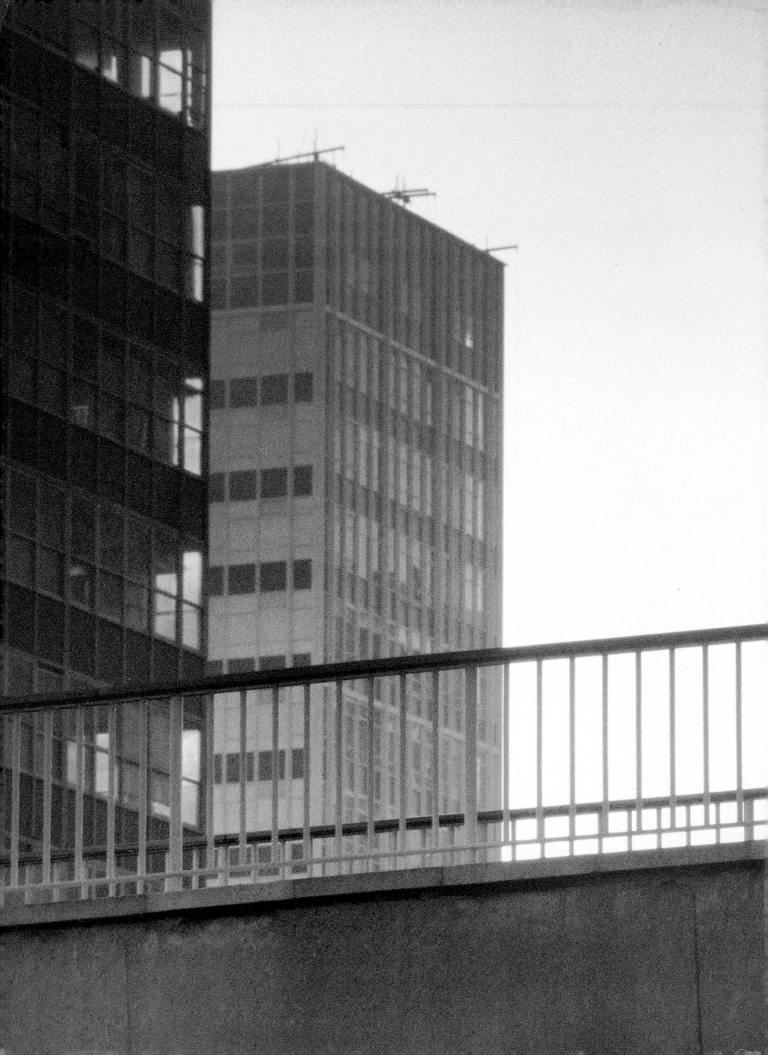

Mineral and source	Function	Mineral and source	Function

Fluoride
A trace element which may be added to water supply. Difficult to get from food sources alone, though found in seafood. Dentists may recommend fluoride toothpastes or tablets.

Important for healthy strong tooth enamel, helps teeth to fight decay.

Phosphorus
Meat, chicken, fish, liver, yeast, cheese, eggs, wheatgerm. Also part of our genetic material – found in every cell.

Good for bones and teeth. Aids utilization of energy from food.

Iodine
Seafood, kelp (seaweed), sea or iodized salt; also in water supply. In some mountain areas, natural water supply has little and will need topping up. A trace element.

Necessary for thyroid gland hormone, properly balanced growth. Deficiency causes goitre, when the thyroid gland swells.

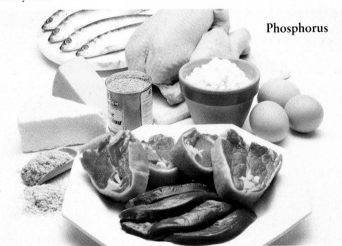

Phosphorus

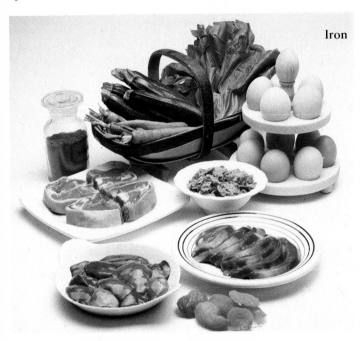

Iron

Potassium
Milk, cheese, seafood, spinach, bananas, butter beans, baked potatoes, dried apricots. Regularly excreted so constant need for replacement.

Insufficiency of both potassium and sodium (see below) can cause loss of muscle tone, problems with nervous system.

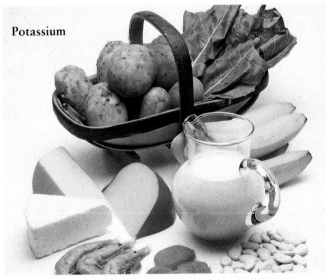

Potassium

Iron
Lamb's liver is the best source (12.6 mg per 85 g (3 oz)). Also chicken liver, meat, dried apricots, cereal products, vegetables, eggs, cocoa, curry powder. Contrary to popular myth spinach, although a good source, is no richer in iron than any other green vegetable. Iron from liver and meat is absorbed more efficiently than iron from other sources; vitamin C increases the body's absorption of iron.

Helps form red corpuscles in blood. Deficiency causes anaemia, lack of energy, fatigue. Women lose iron during pregnancy and lactation, and it is probably the one mineral most women need to top up. Recommended daily intakes vary from 12–18 mg per day; the average diet contains about 12 mg.

Sodium
Salt. Much of what we eat is hidden in processed foods, bread, cereals, flavourings, seafood, dairy products, meat and fish.

Helps balance of fluids, metabolism. A high salt intake may contribute to high blood pressure in some people.

Magnesium
Wholegrain cereals, lentils, green vegetables, beans.

Necessary for metabolism, nerves and muscles.

Sulphur
Eggs, fish, cheese, meat, beans, nuts.

Helps formation of body tissues.

Manganese
Kidneys, lentils, almonds, apricots, watercress, wheatgerm.

Necessary for metabolism, in trace amounts.

Zinc
Meat, cereals, eggs, liver, seafood, wheatgerm. A trace element

Important for sexual maturity and growth, respiration.

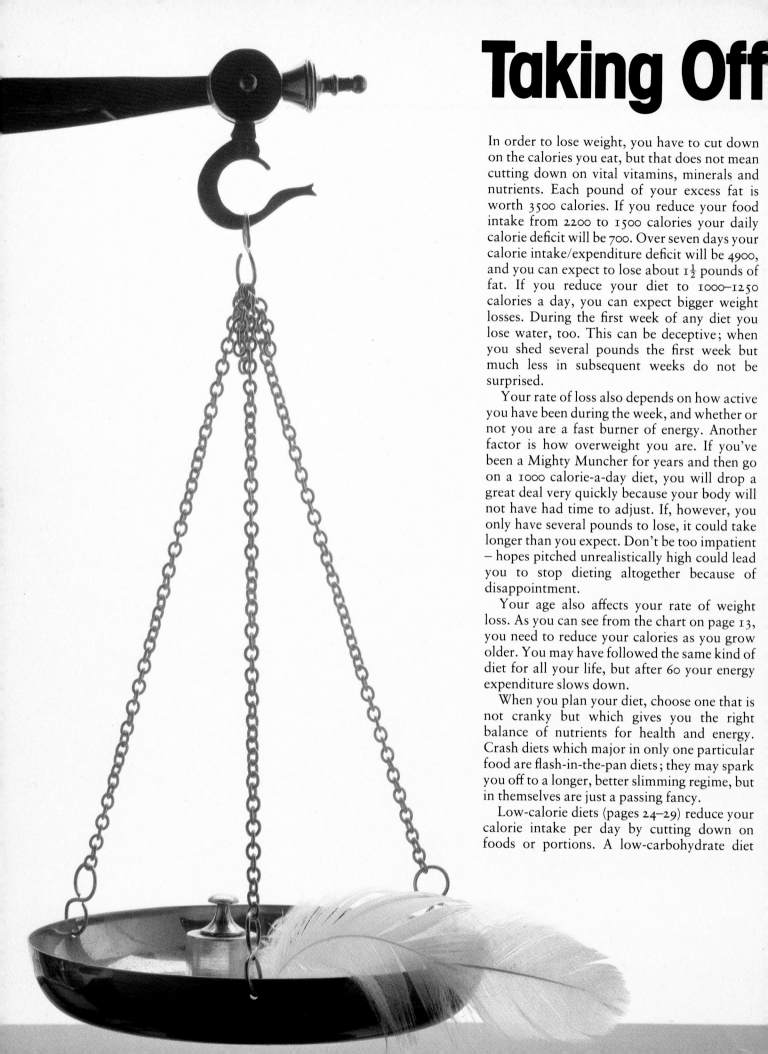

Taking Off

In order to lose weight, you have to cut down on the calories you eat, but that does not mean cutting down on vital vitamins, minerals and nutrients. Each pound of your excess fat is worth 3500 calories. If you reduce your food intake from 2200 to 1500 calories your daily calorie deficit will be 700. Over seven days your calorie intake/expenditure deficit will be 4900, and you can expect to lose about $1\frac{1}{2}$ pounds of fat. If you reduce your diet to 1000–1250 calories a day, you can expect bigger weight losses. During the first week of any diet you lose water, too. This can be deceptive; when you shed several pounds the first week but much less in subsequent weeks do not be surprised.

Your rate of loss also depends on how active you have been during the week, and whether or not you are a fast burner of energy. Another factor is how overweight you are. If you've been a Mighty Muncher for years and then go on a 1000 calorie-a-day diet, you will drop a great deal very quickly because your body will not have had time to adjust. If, however, you only have several pounds to lose, it could take longer than you expect. Don't be too impatient – hopes pitched unrealistically high could lead you to stop dieting altogether because of disappointment.

Your age also affects your rate of weight loss. As you can see from the chart on page 13, you need to reduce your calories as you grow older. You may have followed the same kind of diet for all your life, but after 60 your energy expenditure slows down.

When you plan your diet, choose one that is not cranky but which gives you the right balance of nutrients for health and energy. Crash diets which major in only one particular food are flash-in-the-pan diets; they may spark you off to a longer, better slimming regime, but in themselves are just a passing fancy.

Low-calorie diets (pages 24–29) reduce your calorie intake per day by cutting down on foods or portions. A low-carbohydrate diet (page 30) reduces the amount of sweet and starchy foods you eat. All of these plans involve counting energy units to work out your diet choices. A low-fat diet plan (page 31) cuts down on foods that contain fat or which are fried in fat, allowing you to eat a sensible amount of carbohydrates such as bread and potatoes. All the diet plans ultimately cut down on calories, reducing your energy intake in order to make your body use up its fat stores.

If you find that you dislike counting calories or carbohydrates, and simply want to try to lose weight by cutting down in general and cutting out specific foods, follow the guidelines below. Remember that it isn't just *what* you eat that counts, but *how much*, except for fresh vegetables. And that it's important to include foods from each of the five major food groups – cereals; dairy products; fats; meat, fish and protein; and fruit and vegetables – every day.

Foods to avoid if possible
All alcohol, anything fried, biscuits, butter, cakes, canned fruits in heavy syrup, chocolate, cooking oil, cream, crisps, dried fruit, honey, jam, lard, marmalade, mayonnaise, molasses, nuts, pies, puddings, salad dressing, sugar, sweets, syrup, treacle.

Foods to eat in moderation
Beans, bread, cereals, cheese, margarine, meat, milk, oily fish such as salmon, pasta, pork, potatoes, poultry, rice, sardines, thick soups, tuna.

Foods to eat freely
Bran, consommé, cottage cheese, diet drinks, fresh fruit, fresh vegetables, herbs and spices, kidneys, liver, natural yoghurt, seafood, skimmed milk, unsweetened tea or coffee, white fish.

Cooking Tips

However you plan your diet, the way in which you prepare your food is important. You can make many calorie economies through sensible cooking.
● Grill, do not fry. That way the fat runs off bacon, sausages or chops, instead of congealing around them.
● Cut the fat off meat and the skin from poultry after cooking.
● Fry mincemeat without extra fat and throw away any fat residue by sieving.
● When you cook casseroles, allow time for them to cool – preferably in the fridge overnight. It will then be easy to remove the top layer of fat that forms, before reheating.

● Sauces? Instead of using traditional fat and flour for the roux, use cornflour or arrowroot as a thickener.
● Use skimmed milk instead of ordinary milk.
● Use a low-fat spread instead of butter, yoghurt instead of cream.
● Make your own low-calorie salad dressings to spice up your salads and marinades.

Myths and Pitfalls

Popular theories about dieting seem to be in endless supply, and have been encouraged in recent years by all the fad diets that have come and – in most instances – just as quickly gone. Many of these seem appealing at first glance because they promise rapid weight loss – what you might not realize is that they are often nutritionally imbalanced and rarely offer you the chance to change your eating habits over the long term. The result? You regain all those pounds just a rapidly as you lost them. Let's look at a few of the more common fallacies.

Grapefruit
Diets which insist that you eat half a grapefruit to start every meal because it 'helps to burn off more fat' are misleading. Grapefruit are low in calories, high in vitamin C and therefore a good, convenient food for slimmers. But there is no evidence to substantiate the claim that a grapefruit can speed up your fat/energy conversion rate. The only way you can make your body 'burn' its stores of fat is to take in fewer calories than you expend.

Fat diets
Diets which allow you to eat as much fat and protein as you like, but have you cut out carbohydrates completely, are now being discredited by expert opinion throughout the world. This fad diet is unsafe for your health. Fat can only be broken down completely in the body when carbohydrates are present. Otherwise ketone substances accumulate, producing giddiness and nausea, and giving your breath the smell of rotten apples. (Acetone, sometimes used as a nail varnish remover, is a member of the ketone family.) The ketosis that results is similar to what happens to diabetics if they have a disruption in supplies of insulin. Such a diet is high in saturated fats and cholesterol and, as described by the American Medical Association, 'unscientific and potentially dangerous to health'.

Water
Drinking an excessive amount of water every day will not help your body to get rid of its fat

deposits; your kidneys will simply get rid of the fluid normally. Starting the day with a glass of lemon juice in hot water to 'cleanse your system' is about as effective as grapefruit 'burning up fat'. The Vitamin C in the lemon juice is affected by heat, so whatever vitamin is left will not be contributing much to your daily requirements. There's no harm in drinking water of course; in fact, you should never restrict your intake of water when trying to lose weight.

Deceptive foods

Many foods are obviously loaded with calories, but there are a number of others which are deceptive. Beware of concealed fat in avocado pears, Cheddar, coconuts, cream cheese, French dressing, liver sausage, meat, Parmesan, salami, sausages and Stilton. Concealed sugar lurks in some breakfast cereals, canned soups, dried dates and stem ginger.

It may seem that a lush diet of oysters and steak, cold soups and smoked salmon is better, nutritionally, than a staple fare of meat and potatoes. In the case of watches and motor cars it may be true that an expensive item is of better value than a cheaper one, but it is not necessarily true of foods. You can diet cheaply, simply and well – and still eat foods prepared with taste and imagination.

Slimming Clubs

Group therapy has a good record of success in helping obese people to lose weight. You get support, encouragement and advice, but you have to pay for it. Clubs say that by paying you have a further incentive to stay the course. If you can slim by yourself or with the help of your family, it would seem budget-wise to do so. But if you have a hard time sticking to any diet and weak willpower, then a commercial or local voluntary group could prove helpful.

The advantages are that you can discuss your slimming problems, be weighed and measured, learn new slimming tips and make friends with people who have similar problems. Some drawbacks are that you may feel like a schoolgirl when you do not achieve an adequate weight-loss, grow bored, distrust the lecturers because they do not look slim enough or do not know enough about nutrition.

Some groups are fairly liberal in what diets you follow. Others are very strict and insist that you adhere to a special eating programme. Incentives can vary from small badges to vouchers and scarves. Some groups do exercise sessions at the meetings. All normally have a lecture after your weigh-in.

Aids to Slimming

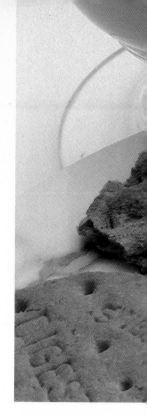

A big slimming-food business has grown up in recent years, aiming to capitalize on the millions of people who are too fat. Some products may be useful as substitutes for higher-calorie foods – slimmers' drinks, for instance – but nothing you can buy will take the place of your own self-control. Nothing you eat can be 'slimming' because all foods contain calories. The best kind of balanced diet helps to re-educate your food habits, so you not only lose unwanted weight, but keep it off, too. Here's a guide to some of the many aids available.

Substitutes

Sweeteners Saccharin tablets are a slimmer's standby, invaluable for adding to hot drinks if you cannot re-educate your palate to do without a tinge of sweetness. Liquid sweeteners, which contain 98 per cent fewer calories than sugar, are useful for cooking. Add them to foods away from the cooker, when they are cooling or cold, to stop any bitter taste. Powder and granulated sweeteners aim to look as much as possible like sugar; some are actual sugar granules coated with saccharin to give extra sweetness; others are concentrated saccharin powders which must be used sparingly. Newer low-calorie, granulated, sugar-free sweeteners have 90 cent fewer calories than sugar, but can be used spoon-for-spoon like sugar, which makes them easier to cope with.

Diet drinks Canned fizzy drinks have almost no calories and are good thirst-quenchers. Low-calorie mixers allow slimmers to have the occasional alcoholic drink and half the normal calories. Low-calorie squashes are also very useful. See drinks guide on pages 34–35.

Low-calorie dressings These are a useful aid to more interesting diets. Low-calorie tomato ketchup is another saving.

Low-calorie spreads A good replacement for butter, giving you more spread on your bread in a calorie-controlled diet. Some taste better than others, so shop around. Processed cheese spreads also give a calorie saving.

Bread Slimmers' breads are lighter, weight for weight, than normal bread, but are usually no different in terms of nutrients. Because they weigh less, their energy value is about half that of ordinary bread. They are worth considering, but not if you eat twice as many slices in an attempt to fill yourself up.

Crispbread Made from wholewheat grains of rye or wheat, usually baked with just a little salt, vegetable oil or water, these are good slimming standbys. As crispbread normally

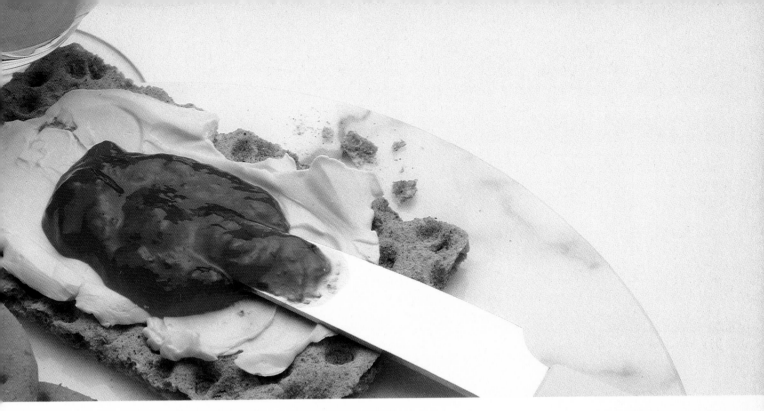

retains the husks of grain, they provide fibre and roughage.

Preserves Low-calorie jams usually have to be kept in the fridge and have about half the calories of ordinary jam.

Canned fruit Unsweetened, natural juice or water instead of syrup means a calorie-saving. A useful substitute, when fresh fruit is not plentiful or available.

Ice cream Slimming ices hardly seem worth bothering about when you can get ordinary ice cream from 30 calories an ounce. The only benefit seems to be that at least you know how many calories they contain, since it's printed on the label.

Milk Skimmed milk and milk with the cream removed are both great slimming aids.

Soups Tins of calorie-conscious soup may prove time-saving, but you can easily make your own diet soups for even fewer calories per serving.

Vegetable cooking spray This provides a less greasy way to pan fry, bake or grill. Since frying is normally forbidden on any slimming diet, this could open up new cooking choices. Spray it on to a cold pan and let the pan warm before adding food; don't be tempted to spray more than the recommended amount.

Meal replacements

Instead of a proper meal, you can have a bar of chocolate, a milkshake, a bowl of soup, a couple of biscuits. They provide you with anything from 125–365 calories and claim to contain added vitamins, minerals, and/or protein. If you do not have time to eat properly then these can make a quick snack, but they should only be used temporarily. Not only are they unsatisfying, but they do not help to re-educate your eating habits into the balanced, healthy eating pattern which will solve your weight problem for life.

'Medical' aids

Appetite reducers Nowadays doctors are less likely to prescribe pills to reduce your appetite unless you are grossly overweight, because of the possibility of dependence and addiction. And taking anything with methyl cellulose in it to make you feel fuller is a waste of time.

Diuretics These make you lose water. Unless you have an illness, which has the effect of making you retain water, you will not help your slimming cause by trying to lose more of it with diuretic pills. And it can be dangerous to lose too much water. The body has its own water-regulating system. You can lose water by sweating – and therefore lose weight – if you go to a Turkish bath or sauna. But you will put it back as soon as you have anything to drink.

Injections Some doctors may give injections of HCG (Human Chorionic Gonadotropin) as a treatment for obesity, together with a very strict diet, but it is not generally accepted by the medical profession.

Body treatments

Slimming garments – from a whole suit to ankle bands – wax treatments and plastic treatments are all sold on the theory that you lose weight as you sweat. But you don't lose fat. You only lose water, which you replace at your very next meal. Slimming 'baths' and slimming 'creams' are equally ineffective.

A selection of low-calorie substitutes: the crispbread is 20 calories, the spread about 105 per 25 g (1 oz), the jam 35 per 25 g (1 oz) and the digestives 40 each. An equivalent snack using full calorie foods would contain about twice the number of calories.

The Diets

The best way to choose a diet plan is to determine your tastes in food, your weaknesses (sweetstuff, for instance), whether you dislike making calculations and how much weight you want to lose. If you're unhappy with the diet you choose and want to change to another, there's nothing to stop you. Be honest when you answer the following questions; using the diet that is right for you makes it that much easier to follow.

– Do you have a lot of weight to lose? If so, you should choose the less stringent type of diet. The low-carbohydrate would be a good choice, because you will need to be on it for quite a while.

● Do you have a sweet tooth? Go for the diet that builds in bonuses and you will be less tempted to cheat.

● Do you like nibbling? Choose the five-meals-a-day plan.

● Do you normally like to eat a lot of bread, potatoes and other starches? Try the low-fat diet.

● Are you always eating out? Go for the low-calorie diet which gives you freedom of choice.

● Are you trying to lose 7–10 pounds? Choose the 1000-calorie diet.

● Do you like the occasional drink? Try a low-calorie diet with a bonus plan.

● Do you enjoy a variety of different kinds of food? Calorie counting would be best: you can eat anything you like as long as you stay within your limit.

● Do you like plenty of fruit and vegetables? Try the low-fat diet.

● Are you worried about your health? Follow the low-fat diet.

The diets which follow give you guidelines for a variety of slimming regimes. Some, such as the 1400-calorie diet and the low-carbohydrate plan, give you suggestions for a complete day's meals; others offer a range of ideas for breakfast, lunch and dinner, allowing you to mix and match. Consult the tables at the back of the book for the calorie, carbohydrate and fat content of foods, and try to devise a programme that suits your tastes and your lifestyle. You may be able to lose weight easily enough if you exercise willpower over the short term, but the only way you'll keep it off once you've lost it is by making sure that you retrain yourself into eating habits that are healthy, sensible, and right for you.

1400 Calories

Limiting yourself to an intake of 1400–1500 calories a day is the maximum for adequate weight loss. Because it is slower than the stringent 1000-calorie plans, this diet is suitable if you want to lose more than 20 pounds, if you lead a very active life, or if you are used to eating big meals and would find the lower-limit plans intolerable. By setting yourself a higher calorie limit, you allow yourself more food and therefore have a better chance of sticking to the diet for a longer period.

Here are three days of menus to kick you off; each day's suggestions add up to approximately 1400 calories. In addition to the foods listed, you have a daily allowance of 560ml (1 pint) skimmed or 280ml (½ pint) normal milk and 25g (1 oz) low-fat spread.

Plan 1

Breakfast
115ml (4 fl oz) orange juice
1 scrambled egg
1 slice wholemeal bread, toasted
coffee or tea

Lunch
small bowl vegetable soup
115g (4 oz) tuna fish with low-calorie dressing
green vegetable salad, as much as you wish
1 slice rye or wholemeal bread
raw carrots
25g (1 oz) Edam cheese
coffee or tea

Dinner
225g (8 oz) raw baked or grilled chicken
85g (3 oz) broccoli
85g (3 oz) green beans
55g (2 oz) boiled macaroni or noodles
green salad with low-calorie dressing
170-g (6-oz) slice melon
coffee or tea

Plan 2

Breakfast
½ grapefruit
25-g (1-oz) portion unsweetened cereal
25g (1 oz) raisins
coffee or tea

Lunch
Sandwich with 1 slice ham, 1 thin slice cheese, lettuce and 2 slices wholemeal bread
any salad vegetables
piece of fruit
coffee or tea

Dinner
170g (6 oz) fish (not fried)
2 small boiled potatoes
115g (4 oz) green vegetables
1 slice wholemeal bread
25g (1 oz) Cheddar cheese
fresh fruit
coffee or tea

Plan 3

Breakfast
140ml (5 fl oz) natural yoghurt
1 apricot
4 walnut halves
coffee or tea

Lunch
55 g (2 oz) corned beef
mixed salad with low-calorie dressing
1 hard-boiled egg
2 crispbreads
115g (4 oz) prunes with 140ml (¼ pint) custard
coffee or tea

Dinner
85g (3 oz) lean roast beef
200-g (7-oz) baked potato
green salad with low-calorie dressing
coffee or tea

It's surprising just how well – and how much – you are allowed to eat on the 1400-calorie diet. Pictured right, Plan 1.

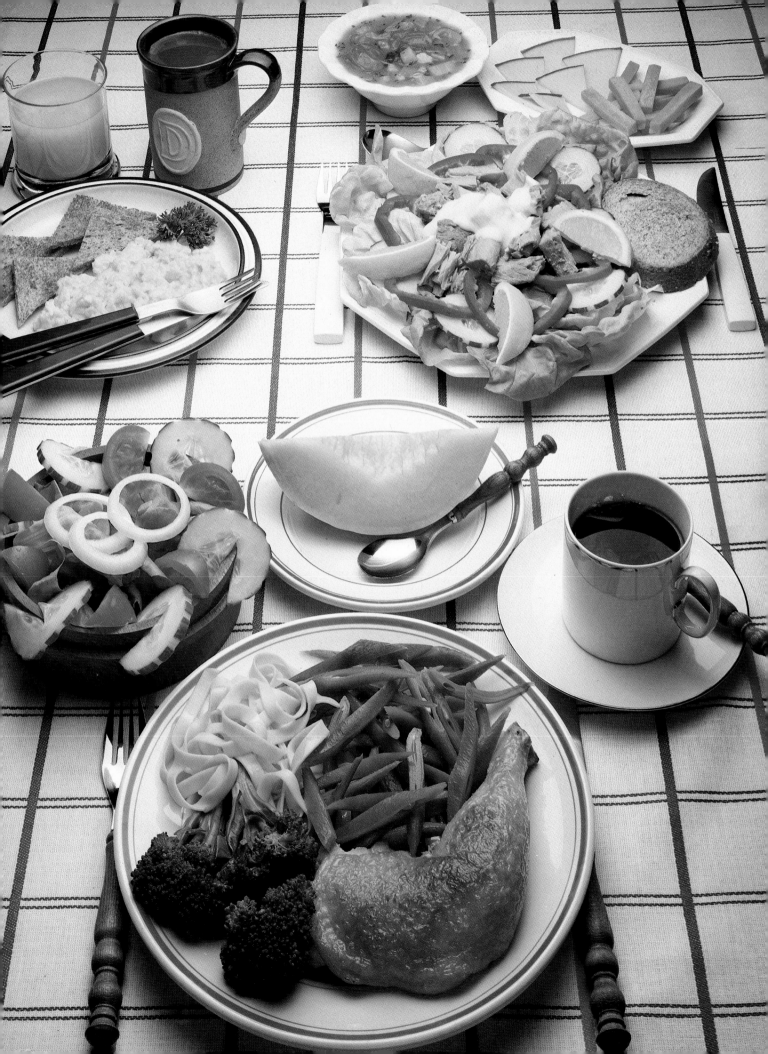

1200-calorie Bonus Plan

We've already seen that one of the best ways to lose weight is to cut down on sweet things altogether, retraining your palate to live without them. But if you can't conquer that craving for these foods, or feel miserable without the occasional drink, this is the diet to choose. It builds in bonuses, so you won't be tempted to cheat. The three menus which follow are good examples of how you can plan your food on this diet; each of them adds up to approximately 1200 calories including a bonus of roughly 200 calories. You also have a daily allowance of 560ml (1 pint) skimmed or 280ml (½ pint) normal milk, which is included, and 25g (1 oz) low-fat spread. Use the list of 100- and 200-calorie bonuses to vary your choice.

Plan 1

Breakfast
115ml (4 fl oz) orange juice
2 scrambled eggs
1 piece bread
coffee or tea

Lunch
1 whole slice tongue
mixed salad with low-calorie
    dressing

Dinner
170g (6 oz) steamed fish
85g (3 oz) green beans
tomato salad with onion

Bonus
170g (6 oz) grapes and 1 glass
    whisky with diet soda

Plan 2

Breakfast
115ml (4 fl oz) orange juice
40g (1½ oz) muesli
coffee or tea

Lunch
cauliflower cheese (use 200g
    (7 oz) cauliflower and 55g
    (2 oz) Edam cheese)

Dinner
115g (4 oz) roast chicken
140-g (5-oz) baked potato
115g (4 oz) carrots
1 fresh pear

Bonus
2 glasses dry white wine *or*
large portion ice cream *or*
35g (1½ oz) chocolate

Plan 3

Breakfast
2 pieces streaky bacon, well
    grilled
1 piece wholemeal bread
coffee or tea

Lunch
115-g (4-oz) beefburger
115g (4 oz) green beans

Dinner
140g (5 oz) grilled lean steak
85g (3 oz) spinach
1 orange

Bonus
2 fruit shortcake biscuits

Bonus choices

The best guide to these is the full calorie counter at the back of the book. Sample bonuses are:

About 100 calories
Small meringue with portion
    ice-cream and fruit
1 glass sweet white wine
1 glass red wine
2 glasses dry sherry
small chocolate-covered roll
1 milk-chocolate wafer biscuit
25g (1 oz) peppermints
2 rich tea biscuits
4 small pieces butterscotch
1 macaroon

About 200 calories
1 small bar chocolate
140g (5 oz) crème caramel
115-g (4-oz) piece pizza
55g (2 oz) chocolate ice cream
    (varies according to
    manufacturer)
560ml (1 pint) beer
1 glass Pimms No. 1 with
    lemonade and fruit
35g (1¼ oz) roasted salted
    peanuts
25g (1 oz) peanut butter
1 chocolate eclair
3 custard cream biscuits

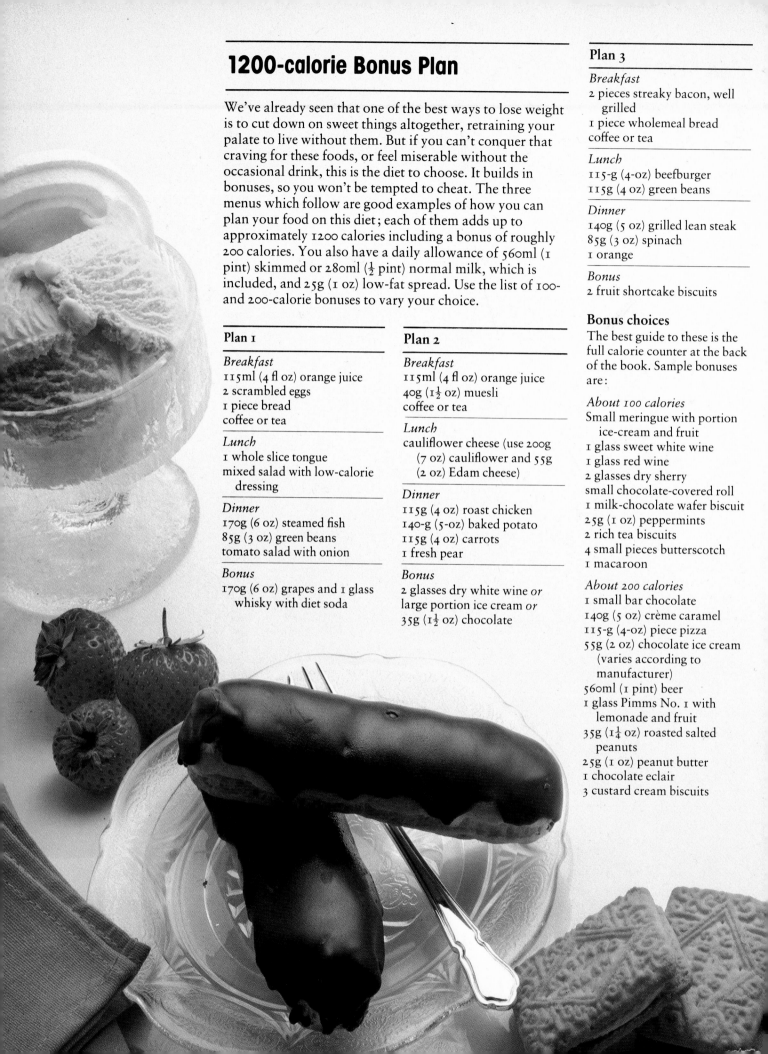

1000 Calories

This is the lowest number of calories a day you should consider for slimming if you want to stay healthy. To save calories, use sugar substitutes and skimmed milk, low-fat spread instead of butter (105 calories instead of 210 per 25g (1 oz)). This diet gives a quicker weight loss than either the low-carbohydrate diet or the previous low-calorie diets. The meals which follow give both the calories of individual dishes and the total for the meal, so you can see what your daily intake will be with various alterations and combinations. There are no extra daily allowances; these have all been built into the meals.

Breakfasts

140ml (5 fl oz) orange juice	45
1 egg, poached or boiled	80
1 slice wholemeal bread with scraping butter	100
Coffee or tea, with milk	20
Total	245
170g (6 oz) grilled kipper fillets	192
1 slice wholemeal bread with low-fat spread	79
coffee or tea with milk	20
Total	291
2 scrambled eggs with little skimmed milk	185
1 crispbread	25
coffee or tea with milk	20
Total	230
130ml (4½ oz) tomato juice	18
25g (1 oz) bran cereal	78
190ml (⅓ pint) skimmed milk	66
coffee or tea with milk	20
Total	182
115g (4 oz) stewed apple with 140ml (5 fl oz) natural yoghurt	115
1 slice wholemeal bread with cheese spread	102
coffee or tea with milk	20
Total	237

Lunches

½ grapefruit	15
55g (2 oz) tuna fish	120
mixed salad	20
yoghurt and lemon juice dressing	30
black coffee	—
Total	185
cauliflower cheese (see page 26)	200
1 apple	40
black coffee	—
Total	240
170-g (6-oz) slice melon	24
115-g (4-oz) fillet of plaice, grilled	108
115g (4 oz) broccoli	20
55g (2 oz) potatoes, boiled	44
Total	196
small bowl clear soup with vegetables	40
225-g (8-oz) piece chicken on the bone, grilled	200
tomato and onion salad with vinegar	28
Total	268
115g (4 oz) honey roast ham	200
mixed salad	20
140g (5 oz) stewed rhubarb with large spoonful natural yoghurt	17
Total	237

Dinners

½ grapefruit	15
115g (4 oz) stewed liver and onions	250
140g (5 oz) plain mashed potatoes	115
apple snow	45
Total	425
425g (15 oz) beef stew	420
apple or pear	40
Total	460
1 large tomato stuffed with cottage cheese	70
140g (5 oz) steamed white fish	135
140g (5 oz) runner beans	20
baked apple stuffed with 25g (1 oz) raisins, ginger, cloves and orange sauce	148
Total	373
mushroom salad with onion and lemon	30
130g (4½ oz) grilled lamb chump chop	200
115g (4 oz) green beans	8
140-g (5-oz) baked potato	120
fresh fruit salad	80
Total	438
125ml (4½ fl oz) tomato juice	18
170g (6 oz) chicken casserole with vegetables	300
85g (3 oz) black grapes	45
Total	363

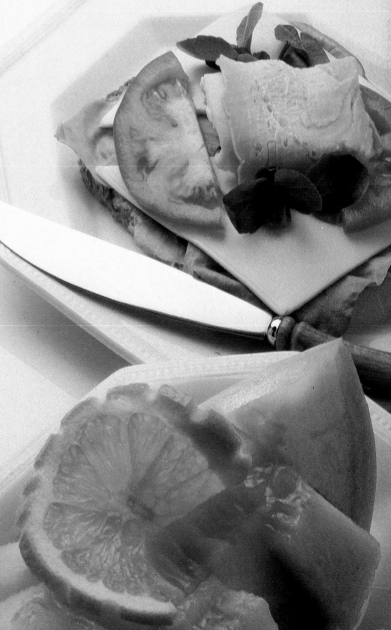

Five Meals a Day (1000 calories)

Slimming experts believe that you will lose weight faster if you divide your daily calorie allowance into five or more smaller meals, rather than two or three big ones. This is because your body uses calories to digest food – and on this diet it will have more opportunities to do so. Although this plan may not be as convenient for those at work all day, it's perfect for women at home, and good for nibblers who prefer the comfort of eating little but often. Your daily allowance is 560ml (1 pint) skimmed or 280ml (½ pint) normal milk.

Breakfasts

115ml (4 fl oz) grapefruit juice
25g (1 oz) bran cereal (with milk from allowance)
coffee or tea
Total : 114

½ grapefruit
1 boiled egg
1 slice wholemeal bread with scraping low-fat spread
coffee or tea
Total : 174

140g (5 oz) haddock, steamed or poached
1 slice slimmer's bread with scraping low-fat spread
coffee or tea
Total : 157

140ml (5 oz) natural yoghurt mixed with 1 apple, sliced
1 rye or wheat crispbread with scraping low-fat spread
coffee or tea
Total : 157

2 pieces streaky bacon, well grilled
45ml (3 tbs) canned tomatoes
1 slice slimmer's bread
coffee or tea
Total : 135

Extra meals (mid-morning or evening)

55g (2 oz) green grapes
2 rye crispbreads with 25g (1 oz) curd cheese and slices of cucumber, tomato
Total : 132

1 tangerine
115g (4 oz) cottage cheese
1 crispbread
green salad with low-calorie dressing
Total : 193

mug hot chocolate (55ml (2 fl oz) milk, 10 ml (2 tsp) drinking chocolate and water)
1 pear
1 slice wholemeal bread with scraping low-fat spread
Total : 181

170-g (6-oz) slice melon
small cup clear soup
1 slice bread with scraping low-fat spread
Total : 141

small bowl vegetable soup
croutons made from 1 slice slimmer's bread
1 orange
Total : 135

lemon tea
1 banana
open sandwich with 1 slice slimmer's bread, scraping low-fat spread, 1 mashed sardine and cucumber slices
Total : 197

1 crispbread spread with 5ml (1 tsp) sweetened condensed milk, quartered apple and 5ml (1 tsp) raisins
Total : 100

115g (4 oz) stewed rhubarb mixed with 140ml (5 oz) natural yoghurt
Total : 81

Lunches

85g (3 oz) cottage cheese
25g (1 oz) lean ham
2 chopped walnut halves
green salad
Total : 157

2 chicken drumsticks, grilled
mixed salad with low-calorie dressing
Total : 242

170-g (6-oz) baked potato with 55g (2 oz) cottage cheese and chives, seasoning, onion
Total : 195

85g (3 oz) prawns
115g (4 oz) new potatoes
25g (1 oz) shredded cabbage, carrot, red and green pepper slices with low-calorie dressing
Total : 250

1 poached egg on spinach
2 plums
Total : 137

Dinners

1 grilled lamb's kidney
1 grilled piece bacon
1 grilled tomato
55g (2 oz) grilled mushrooms
Total : 102

140g (5 oz) baked cod, stuffed with breadcrumbs, mustard, pinch herbs, 25g (1 oz) mushrooms
140g (5 oz) green beans
Total : 211

bowl slimmer's vegetable soup
2-egg omelette with herbs
Total : 200

115g (4 oz) canned salmon
mixed salad with low-calorie dressing
Total : 238

85g (3 oz) lean lamb chunks on skewer
1 tomato
slices green pepper
few mushrooms
Total : 244

170-g (6-oz) joint of chicken
140g (5 oz) cooked cabbage
55g (2 oz) carrots
Total : 182

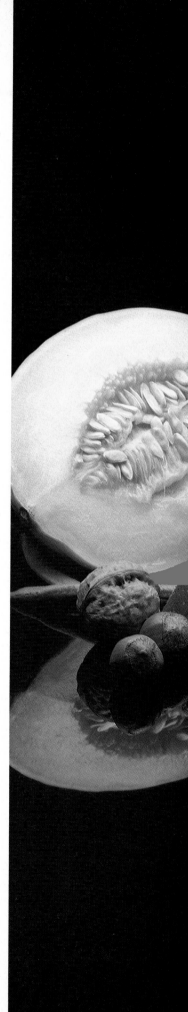

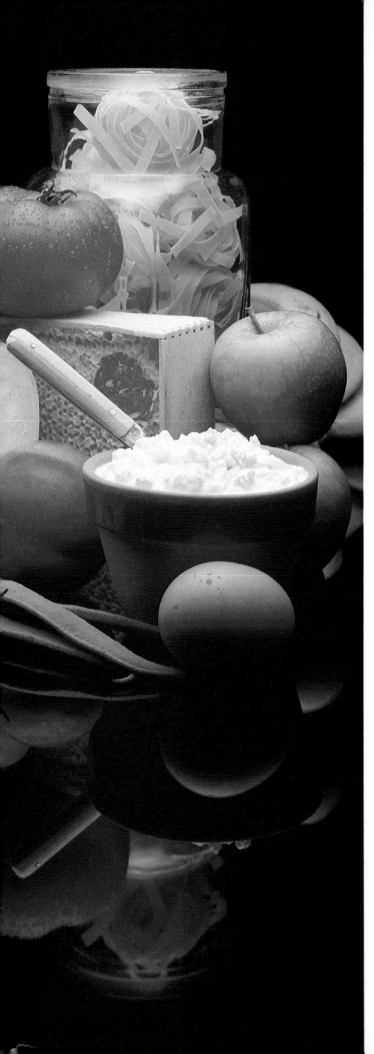

Vegetarian (1000 calories)

If you prefer not to eat meat, here is a special diet plan which provides choices for 200, 300 and 400 calorie meals. One meal from each of the categories, together with a 280ml (½ pint) skimmed milk allowance, will total 1000 calories a day. In addition to milk, your daily allowance includes 25g (1 oz) low-fat spread or 15g (½ oz) butter or margarine and 1 slice wholemeal bread or 2 crispbreads. Any bread or crispbread listed in the meals is in addition to the allowance.

Most vegetables are wonderfully low in calories as long as you don't fry them – boil or steam them, or braise them in a little stock. In addition to the meals given below, you can eat freely from any vegetables such as artichokes, asparagus, broccoli, brussels sprouts, cabbage, carrots, cauliflower, celery, green beans, lettuce, mushrooms, onions, radishes, spinach, tomatoes, turnips and watercress.

200 calories

2-egg omelette (plain, herb or tomato) made with 9g (⅓ oz) low-fat spread

---

2 thin slices slimmer's bread, toasted, with scraping low-fat spread
140g (5 oz) baked beans

25g (1 oz) raisins
20g (¾ oz) nuts

170-g (6-oz) baked potato, filled with 25g (1 oz) cottage cheese and chopped herbs

---

2 large baked apples, sweetened with 25g (1 oz) honey and cinnamon

---

1 corn on the cob with 25g (1 oz) low-fat spread

300 calories

risotto with 55g (2 oz) rice, celery, onion, mushrooms, tomatoes and 50g (1¾ oz) Cheddar cheese

---

green pepper stuffed with 55g (2 oz) rice, 40g (1½ oz) grated cheese and onion
115g (4 oz) fresh pineapple

115-g (4-oz) piece cheese and tomato pizza

---

average portion ratatouille
small potato and cheese pancake

---

cole slaw with 55g (2 oz) Edam cheese, 2 walnuts and low-calorie dressing

fresh beansprouts, cooked with mushrooms, onion, celery and a few almonds with sweet and sour sauce
170g (6 oz) baked egg custard

400 calories

haricot or kidney beans baked with tomatoes, onion and 25g (1 oz) Edam cheese
115-g (4-oz) baked potato

---

small bowl bortsch
1 poached egg with spinach and 25g (1 oz) grated cheese

---

macaroni cheese (55g (2 oz) macaroni; 25g (1 oz) cheese)
170-g (6-oz) slice melon

115-g (4-oz) cottage cheese
1 peach
1 banana
salad vegetables
140ml (5 oz) natural yoghurt with 15g (½ oz) raisins and 2 walnut halves

---

vegetable soup
170-g (6-oz) baked potato
mixed salad
170-g (6-oz) slice melon

Vegetarian foods, left, offer a wide variety of low-calorie ideas for slimmers.

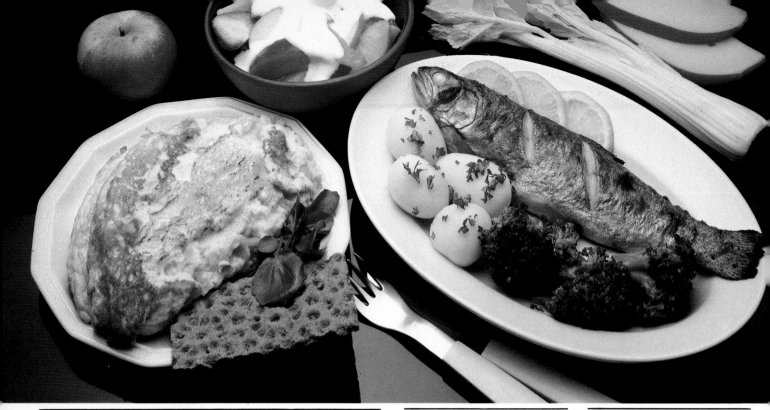

Low-carbohydrate

A diet which restricts sweet and starchy foods, this is a well-tried favourite method of slimming. The Carbohydrate Unit, equivalent to five grammes of carbohydrate, is a convenient way to calculate your intake, which should be no more than ten CUs a day. Sounds simple? It is, but you can go wrong and find your diet is unsuccessful if you think that you can eat *anything* other than carbohydrates. You need to restrict your all-round calorie intake, from whatever source of food. This means keeping an eye on the alternatives. For instance, eating a lot more hard cheese instead of bread could mean you stop losing weight. Hard cheese is a high-fat, high-calorie food; choose cottage or curd cheese instead.

This sort of diet gives you a daily calorie intake of about 1500, which does shed the pounds, but rather more slowly than a 1000-calorie plan. It often works well if you have a considerable amount of weight to lose, and is a good diet if you do not like counting calories and are not a between-meals nibbler.

The menus which follow give you ideas for three days. Look up foods in the chart on pages 76–78 to work out other meal plans. Don't remove all the carbohydrates from your meals, or you won't be eating a balanced diet. Although an o indicates a negligible amount of carbohydrates and, in theory, this should mean you can eat as much as you want, do remember the pitfalls. The best carbohydrates to restrict are the sweet ones, such as cakes, biscuits and chocolate, rather than fruit, vegetables and whole cereals. Spread your carbohydrate units over the day – a few units at each meal – and you'll feel better and have more freedom of choice. And remember that drinks have to be counted, too. Only water, tea and coffee, without milk and sugar, are freely allowed. Daily allowance is 280ml ($\frac{1}{2}$ pint) milk – $2\frac{1}{2}$ CUs.

Plan 1

140ml (5 oz) natural yoghurt with 115g (4 oz) fresh fruit	$4\frac{1}{2}$
1 crispbread lightly buttered	1
coffee or tea	0
2-egg ham omelette	0
1 apple	2
liver casserole	0
115g (4 oz) courgettes	0
brussels sprouts	0
canteloupe melon	0

Plan 2

115ml (4 oz) unsweetened orange juice	2
1 boiled egg	0
1 slice slimmer's bread, lightly buttered	$1\frac{1}{2}$
coffee or tea	0
115g (4 oz) cottage cheese with mixed salad	0
1 medium-sized mandarin	1
1 dry sherry	2
85g (3 oz) roast meat	0
cauliflower	0
french beans	0
2 plums	1

Plan 3

$\frac{1}{2}$ grapefruit	$\frac{1}{2}$
2 pieces grilled bacon	0
1 slice wholemeal bread, lightly buttered	2
coffee or tea	0
braised beef	0
115g (4 oz) green beans	0
115g (4 oz) cauliflower	0
55g (2 oz) Camembert cheese	0
1 crispbread, starch reduced	$\frac{1}{2}$
115ml (4 fl oz) tomato juice	1
grilled fish	0
broccoli	0
85g (3 oz) new potatoes	3
piece celery with 1 starch-reduced crispbread and 55g (2 oz) Edam cheese	$\frac{1}{2}$

A tempting array of meals you can eat on a low-carbohydrate (above left) or low-fat (above right) diet.

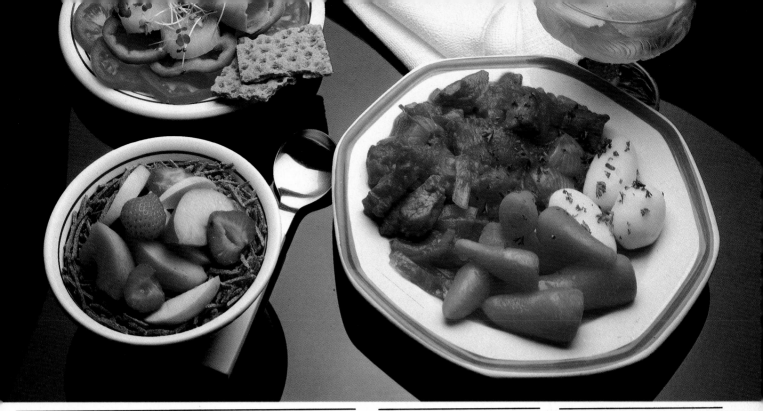

Low-fat

Fats are a high source of calories in your diet, almost twice that of protein and carbohydrate, so if you reduce the amount you eat, you automatically cut down on your own surplus body fat. Of course, that doesn't mean you can drink lots of high-calorie wine and eat loaves of bread every day. You need to be sensible about the alternative foods you consume. Rough starches are certainly allowed, especially the wholemeal cereals and potatoes which provide both vitamins and fibre, the bulk that stops you feeling so hungry.

This diet can be of particular benefit to your health since, as we have seen, doctors believe our fat intake is currently much higher than it needs to be. The meal ideas listed here should get you started; consult the list at the back of the book for high-, medium- and low-fat foods. Allow yourself 280ml ($\frac{1}{2}$ pint) skimmed milk and 15g ($\frac{1}{2}$ oz) low-fat spread per day. (Butter and hard margarines are out.) Try using vegetable spray on your pans instead of conventional frying fats. Watch your cheeses: cottage cheese is lowest in fat, then curd; cream cheese is highest, so avoid it. Edam and Camembert have less fat than most other cheeses. You can eat rice and pasta, but only with low-fat sauces, three portions of fruit per day and unlimited amounts of vegetables. If you want a snack between meals, choose a small carton of natural yoghurt or some raw vegetables like carrots.

Menu 1

Breakfast
bran cereal with fresh fruit or
    canned prunes
coffee or tea

Lunch
salad of tomato, celery heart,
    cress, green pepper and 55g
    (2 oz) lean ham, with low-
    calorie dressing
1 slice bread or crispbread
fresh fruit
coffee or tea

Dinner
veal paprika
boiled carrots
boiled potatoes
green salad
fruit sorbet
coffee or tea

Menu 2

Breakfast
portion smoked haddock
1 slice bread
stewed apple
coffee or tea

Lunch
1 grilled hamburger
fruit and vegetable salad with
    low-calorie dressing
portion ice cream
coffee or tea

Dinner
liver and onion casserole
green vegetables
slice melon
coffee or tea

Menu 3

Breakfast
small can baked beans in
    tomato sauce
1 slice bread, toasted
1 glass orange juice
coffee or tea

Lunch
115g (4 oz) chicken, skin
    removed
green salad with low-calorie
    dressing
1 slice wholemeal bread
1 piece fruit
coffee or tea

Dinner
risotto
soft or other fresh fruit
coffee or tea

Menu 4

Breakfast
oat porridge
unsweetened grapefruit juice
coffee or tea

Lunch
cheese salad sandwich on
    wholemeal bread
fresh fruit
coffee or tea

Dinner
spaghetti bolognese (use 55g
    (2 oz) pasta and 115g (4 oz)
    minced beef)
baked peach with natural
    yoghurt
coffee or tea

Social Diet

If there's one thing that's sure to test any slimmer's willpower to the limits, it is eating out socially, or having people round for meals in your own home – although that is at least more controllable. 'Do have another drink,' says one hostess. 'You simply must try my new pudding,' says another, giving your conscience a tweak. And if you have the kind of job that means having business lunches and drinking, you could be faced with delicious choices in smart restaurants. So how can you carry on with your diet, not become a bore, and stay sociable? Here's how to meet some of the challenges.

Drinks
Remember that wines and alcohol are just as full of calories as food. See the drinks list on pages 34–35 for choices. You can't stand around at parties without a drink in your hand, so ask for a spritzer (white wine mixed with soda or fizzy mountain spring mineral water). A long, diluted drink is best, with ice-cubes, because you can sip it slowly and spin it out longer. If you're being very strict, a slimline tonic poured over ice-cubes with a slice of lemon looks convincingly like a gin-and-tonic. Low-calorie ginger ale on ice looks like Scotch on the rocks. If you think it sounds a bit 'soft' to ask for a diet drink, have one shot of alcohol – and keep on filling up with the mixer. Your glass looks full all the time.

Cocktail and buffet parties
All those crisps, dips, nuts and hors d'oeuvres can send your calorie-count soaring. Remove yourself from the food corner of any room and keep your hands occupied, with drink and bag, so that you'll find it more difficult to reach for the nuts.

Self-service buffet parties give you the chance to take what you want. Slices of meat or poultry are fine; there's bound to be salad, but go easy on the mayonnaise. Skip the roll and butter. If you cannot bear to miss out on the desserts, have the smallest of helpings to satisfy your taste-buds. But avoid cheesecake at all costs because it is enormously high in calories. A meringue is a better choice, surprisingly!

Dinner parties
These are most difficult when you are at somebody else's house, because you are faced with a meal which the hostess has cooked for you, without alternatives, and it would seem rude to refuse a helping. The only thing you can do is go prepared. Eat the minimal amount beforehand: work out how many calories you think you will eat at dinner, then save them from meals earlier in the day. Don't have second helpings, and don't indulge in both cheese and the pudding. Sip your wine, so your glass doesn't need much replenishing.

Your own dinner parties are easy because you can whip up some fairly low-calorie but gourmet-style meals and stock up on slimmers' drinks. There's no reason why your guests have to eat bland, tasteless food because you are on a diet. Home-made soups give plenty of room for invention and make a delicious first course. You don't need to add cream. In casseroles, you can use emulsified vegetables such as onions and carrots as the thickener. Camembert and Edam are lower in calories than other cheeses. Buy yourself a good dieter's cookbook, but test the recipes in advance.

Eating out
When you're in a restaurant the choice is yours, so choose wisely. It is so easy to be seduced by the huge menu, by what the people at the next table are eating, or by the sweet trolly parked close to your left ear. First ask the waiter to remove the bread and rolls and butter from the table – if your companion doesn't mind! Otherwise, make sure it is not too close to you. With butter at 210 calories an ounce, it just isn't worth filling yourself up before the meal even begins.

Pick your way through the menu as if through a minefield. As you are paying for service as well as food, have the food as you want it. For instance, you can ask the waiter to serve the vegetables without butter.

For a first course, you could have fruit or tomato juice, grapefruit, melon, consommé, or even oysters. The ones to avoid? Rich creamy soups or soups with cheese and bread, such as French Onion Soup. Pâté is high in fat and lethal to any diet; with toast and butter it could be as much as 850 calories. Mayonnaise dishes – prawn cocktail, egg mayonnaise – are not such a good idea; nor are dishes with a pastry or pizza base. Smoked salmon is about 40 calories an ounce and portions are usually wafer thin, so you could be quite safe with it as a starter . . . except for the brown bread and butter which usually accompanies it. Half an avocado with oil and vinegar is a very high-calorie choice. Melon and Parma ham, smoked eel, any non-creamy, non-buttery soup, or dish which is not fried, can be considered.

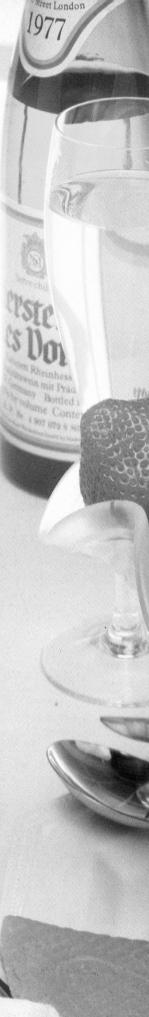

For your main course, a simple grilled dish is probably the best. Avoid pizzas, fatty lamb cutlets, mixed grills, anything fried in batter, chips, pies and puddings made with suet pastry, pork, lasagne. Salads are fine, so long as they are not dripping in high-calorie dressing, fried bread croûtons, masses of grated cheese and pieces of bacon. Kebabs are a better bet than Moussaka, braised kidneys rather than roast duck. A lean piece of grilled fillet steak, grilled chicken (don't eat the skin), or sweet and sour chicken would be better than big fry-ups.

Fresh fruit, without cream, or fresh fruit salad, is a good dessert choice for dieters. If you're carbohydrate counting, though, be careful. A small portion of soft fruit is about 1½CUs. Sorbet or ice-cream are better than Rum Baba and Chocolate Cherry Cake, at least in calories. Avoid cheesecake, baked sponge puddings, rich chocolate-cream concoctions, apple strudel, fritters fried in batter, or fruit with crumble topping. Crème caramel, peach melba, oranges sliced in caramel sauce and frothy light Zabaglione can be considered. Say no to cheese and biscuits. Irish coffee is about 350 calories, so don't indulge.

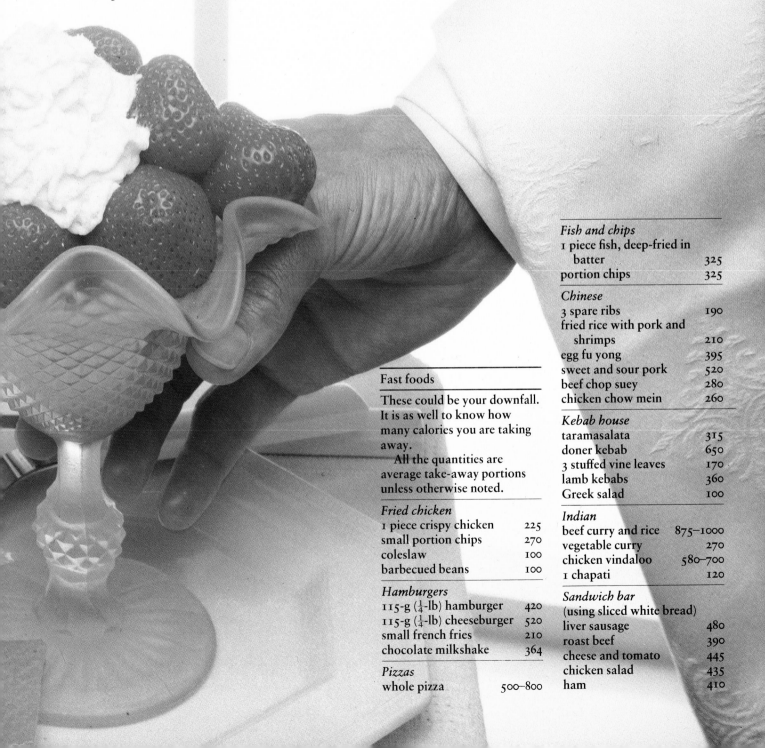

Fish and chips

1 piece fish, deep-fried in batter	325
portion chips	325

Chinese

3 spare ribs	190
fried rice with pork and shrimps	210
egg fu yong	395
sweet and sour pork	520
beef chop suey	280
chicken chow mein	260

Kebab house

taramasalata	315
doner kebab	650
3 stuffed vine leaves	170
lamb kebabs	360
Greek salad	100

Indian

beef curry and rice	875–1000
vegetable curry	270
chicken vindaloo	580–700
1 chapati	120

Sandwich bar
(using sliced white bread)

liver sausage	480
roast beef	390
cheese and tomato	445
chicken salad	435
ham	410

Fast foods

These could be your downfall. It is as well to know how many calories you are taking away.

All the quantities are average take-away portions unless otherwise noted.

Fried chicken

1 piece crispy chicken	225
small portion chips	270
coleslaw	100
barbecued beans	100

Hamburgers

115-g (¼-lb) hamburger	420
115-g (¼-lb) cheeseburger	520
small french fries	210
chocolate milkshake	364

Pizzas

whole pizza	500–800

A CALORIE-COUNTED DRINKS GUIDE

Counting the calories can be a bit deceptive, since different brands have different calorific values. Cider and beer, in particular, vary considerably according to manufacturer. The figures given here are average amounts.

DRINKS	CALORIES	AMOUNT
NON-ALCOHOLIC DRINKS		
Bottled spring waters, mineral waters (e.g. Evian, Perrier), soda water	0	
Black coffee	Negligible	
Lemon tea without sugar	Negligible	
Low-calorie diet drinks and squashes	Negligible	
Tea or coffee with 30 ml (2 tbs) skimmed milk	10	170 ml (6 fl oz)
Tea or coffee with 30 ml (2 tbs) normal milk	20	170 ml (6 fl oz)
Tomato juice	20	140 ml (5 fl oz)
Peppermint cordial	25	30 ml (1 fl oz)

DRINK	CALORIES	AMOUNT
Tonic water	25	140 ml (5 fl oz)
Dry ginger ale	30	140 ml (5 fl oz)
Tomato and vegetable juice	30	140 ml (5 fl oz)
Lemonade	30	140 ml (5 fl oz)
Orange squash (concentrate)	30	30 ml (1 fl oz)
Lime juice cordial (concentrate)	32	30 ml (1 fl oz)
Blackcurrant drink (concentrate)	32.5	15 ml ($\frac{1}{2}$ fl oz)
Lemon Barley	35	30 ml (1 fl oz)
Grapefruit juice (unsweetened)	45	140 ml (5 fl oz)
Orange juice (unsweetened)	45	140 ml (5 fl oz)
Tea with 30 ml (1 fl oz) milk and 10 ml (2 tsp) sugar	48	170 ml (6 fl oz)
Coffee with 30 ml (1 fl oz) milk and 10 ml (2 tsp) sugar	48	170 ml (6 fl oz)

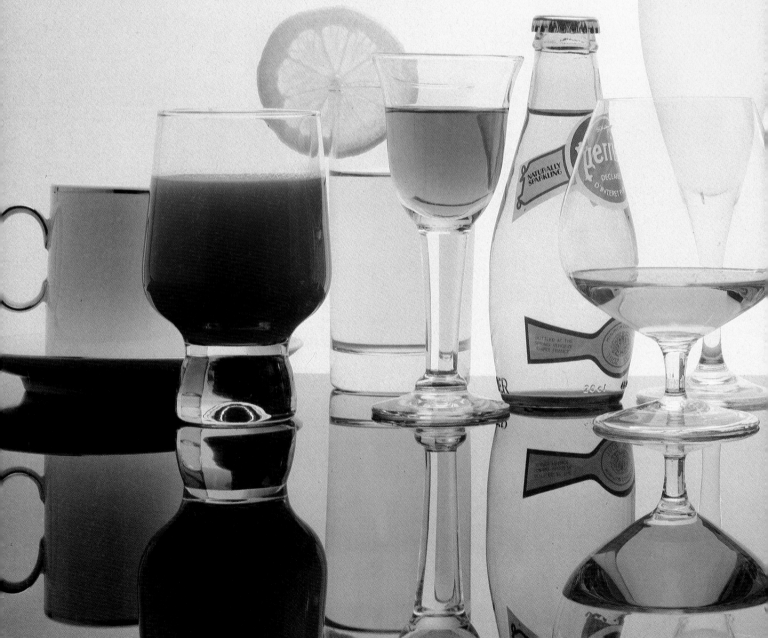

DRINK	CALORIES	AMOUNT
Cola	55	140 ml (5 fl oz)
Iced black coffee with 40 g (1½ oz) ice cream	72	170 ml (6 fl oz)
Pineapple juice (unsweetened)	75	140 ml (5 fl oz)
Skimmed milk	200	560 ml (1 pt)
Milk (normal)	370	560 ml (1 pt)

ALCOHOLIC DRINKS

DRINK	CALORIES	AMOUNT
Spirits (gin, whisky, vodka at 70 proof, rum, bourbon, brandy)	63	30 ml (1 fl oz)
Dry sherry	66	55 ml (2 fl oz)
Dry vermouth	68	55 ml (2 fl oz)
Medium sherry	68	55 ml (2 fl oz)
Vermouth rosso	75	55 ml (2 fl oz)
Dry white wine	76	110 ml (4 fl oz)
Dry red wine	76	110 ml (4 fl oz)

DRINK	CALORIES	AMOUNT
Sweet sherry	78	55 ml (2 fl oz)
Rosé wine	80	110 ml (4 fl oz)
Vermouth rosé	80	55 ml (2 fl oz)
Liquers	80	30 ml (1 fl oz)
Vermouth bianco	86	55 ml (2 fl oz)
Sparkling white wine	88	110 ml (4 fl oz)
Port	90	55 ml (2 fl oz)
Sweet white wine	108	110 ml (4 fl oz)
Stout	110	280 ml (½ pt)
Beer	75–135	280 ml (½ pt)
Cider	100–200	280 ml (½ pt)
Barley wine	255	280 ml (½ pt)

Helping Your Willpower

Psychologists have found the key to changing your eating habits. It's a concept in weight control called behaviour therapy and it is based on the theory that eating too much for your energy requirements is behaviour that you learn. From the cradle we respond to eating cues; mothers reward the baby who finishes its bottle with a warm smile and a kiss; a biscuit helps to allay the pain of a fall; a piece of chocolate is earned by the toddler who responds well to toilet-training. That's how we learn to eat without being hungry. Then, as adults, we find that we are eating because we feel bored, lonely or sad, or because it's 'lunchtime' or it's sociable.

Behaviour therapy applies psychological principles to change those habits that led to your being overweight in the first place. Similar programmes are often used to help people stop smoking. Try the suggestions below. Each of them could help you to learn to eat less.

● Observe your eating patterns. You won't be successful in changing them until you actually realize what they are. Try to keep a notebook or diary and write down the time you eat, what you eat and where you are at the time. You could discover that you eat almost without knowing it, while watching television, or as you cook.

● Count calories for a while. Add up all the calories you have eaten on a typical day. Then you can see how much you will need to cut down to lose weight.

● Slow down. The idea is to eat a bit less but enjoy it all the more. Eat your food like a gourmet, savouring every bite. Serve fish and poultry on the bone to make them harder to eat quickly. It takes about 20 minutes from when you start eating for your stomach to signal to your brain that you are full; if you stretch out your meal you could end up feeling fuller on less.

● Don't feel you have to eat everything on your plate. It won't go to the starving millions, only into the garbage. Cut down your portion sizes and use a smaller plate so you won't feel cheated.

● Keep all food in the kitchen so you won't be faced with nibbles in other places. Don't combine eating with any other activity.

● Think up alternatives to nibbling. Instead of lunch, why not take a nap if you're at home. Many of us could do with more sleep and it will make you feel refreshed. If you knit while watching television, you cannot be using your hands to reach for crisps or other nibbles.

● Treat each snack as if it were a meal. Take a knife and fork to an apple. Set the table. Consciously control what you eat.

● Make sure the only nibbles easily available are the low-calorie ones such as carrots, cucumber, celery, radishes, green pepper, mushrooms, cauliflower, lettuce etc.

● Delay eating. Don't eat that snack until after you have done something else, whether it is

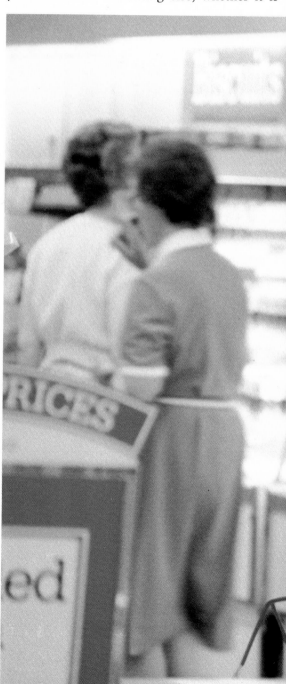

finishing a job or calling a friend.

● Save up food from one meal to another – for instance, save bread from breakfast and have it as a snack mid-morning or later in the day. No food is forbidden – just controlled. Think that, and you won't be so obsessive about denying yourself.

● Do not reward yourself with food – that could well have been the start of obesity problems. Instead, devise leisure incentives – a new book, a trip to the theatre, some new clothes. Or give a certain amount of money to charity for every pound you lose.

● Dull your appetite before a cocktail party with a bowl of clear soup, or some raw vegetables.

● Shop wisely. Make a list first and carry only the amount of money you need for the food on the list. Buy for now, not for next week. Try to stop impulse buying, 'just this once'. Shop after eating – you'll buy more when you're hungry – and not when you're depressed.

● Be resolute if you're cooking for a family. Fried foods, heavy dressings and rich desserts aren't good for them either.

● Look at your lost weight. Tell a friend you've lost five pounds and it means almost nothing. But hold a five-pound bag of sand or flour and you can see how heavy it is.

● Make a list of the differences you notice as you lose weight – receiving compliments from strangers, not being told there's nothing available in your size, being able to wear a bikini for the first time in years.

● Don't be hard on yourself if you don't lose as much a week as you think you should. Set yourself more modest goals – one or two pounds a week instead of seven.

● Share dieting with a friend and bolster each other up. Or join a slimming club for support.

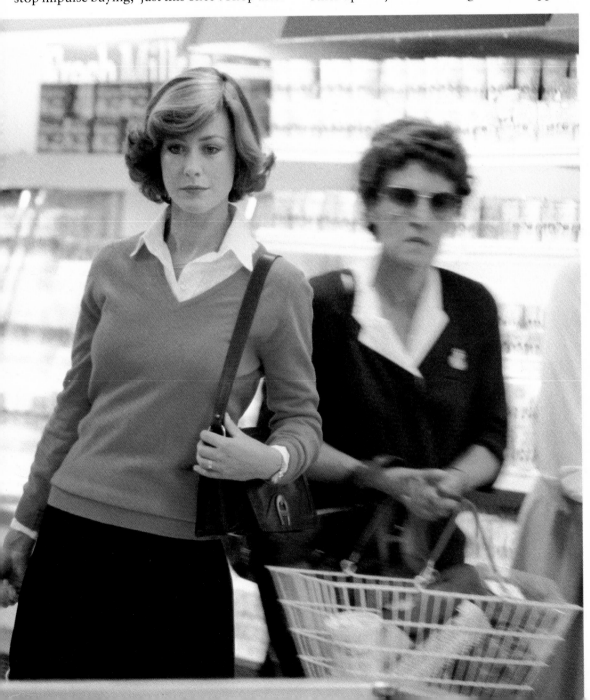

Be careful when you shop for food – a temptation resisted in the supermarket is one less to worry about at home.

Moving into Top Gear

What is the most important thing you can do for your health? Most of the world's top experts agree that keeping your weight within reasonable limits and taking physical exercise have to be top priorities. The only trouble about exercise is getting started! We all mean to do it, one day, but somehow or other we never seem to have the time. What we should remember is that it's important to *make* the time in order to keep fit. Remember, too, that exercise is an invaluable aid to slimming. In addition to burning calories and toning your muscles as you lose that extra fat, it can, surprisingly, even *reduce* your appetite. Dieters have always been afraid that taking more exercise would make them want to eat more, but recent studies with overweight women in the United States show different results. The body senses low blood sugar as an emergency and when your body knows it lacks fuel (from food) you get the urge to eat. But exercise causes the body to release stored food in the fat cells, turning off the hunger alarm. Exercise also causes the body to release adrenalin, which has the effect on the brain of decreasing feelings of hunger. By increasing your level of activity, regularly, you may even speed up your metabolism in general, say the experts. Greater blood flow to the thyroid gland, caused by exercise, can stimulate it to produce more hormones to speed up the rate at which the body burns up calories.

Besides its physical benefits, taking more exercise in order to stay fit has an uplifting effect on your morale. It helps to banish stress, encourages healthy sleep and aids concentration. Medically, it reduces your risk of heart disease, chest trouble, arthritis and high blood pressure. Make your body work for a living, and it will repay you with increased vigour and delight. Give in to a sedentary non-active life, and your years will weigh heavily.

How fit are you?

As the saying goes, if you don't want to lose it, use it. The body deteriorates if it is not used fully enough. Like a creaky old machine that needs oiling, it splutters and grumbles, dawdles along. If you have ever been in a hospital and had to stay in bed for a week or two, you will know it takes some time before you are fully mobile again. You have to learn to walk and build up your strength slowly, re-adjusting to movement and exercise.

There are three major fitness factors: suppleness, strength and stamina. Test yourself in each of these areas to see how fit you really are. Weight also plays a part – heavy people are generally less fit than those who maintain their ideal weight.

Suppleness

Being supple means easy, graceful movement, flexible joints and active, well-toned muscles. If you can't bend down without groaning, or find it hard to reach a high shelf or do up your bra, you'll need to do stretching exercises, known as calesthenics, to increase your flexibility. Lack of suppleness could also lead to poor posture and back pain.

To test your suppleness, bend at the waist and try to touch the floor with the tips of your fingers. Or lie on your back and hook your feet under the bed, a cupboard or a heavy chair, arms straight at your sides or vertically in the air. Keeping both arms and legs straight, sit up slowly, then return to the floor. If you find this easy to do, you're quite supple; if you can do it 10 times, you have good stamina as well.

Strength

This is the area where women are traditionally weakest. Bear in mind that muscular strength does not necessarily mean the ability to lift heavy weights – and you don't have to prove your femininity by being feeble! It's more to do with good, firm muscle tone. When you don't use your muscles they grow weak and thin; when you exercise them properly they help take up slack flesh – a flabby stomach, for instance – and prevent poor posture and back problems. Women can be strong without developing bulky muscles, because muscle size is related to hormone levels.

To test your strength, do sit-ups (page 50) for one minute. If you can only do five, you're not very strong; if you can do as many as 25, you're quite strong, and have good stamina as well. If you feel the strain, stop immediately; this is not an endurance test.

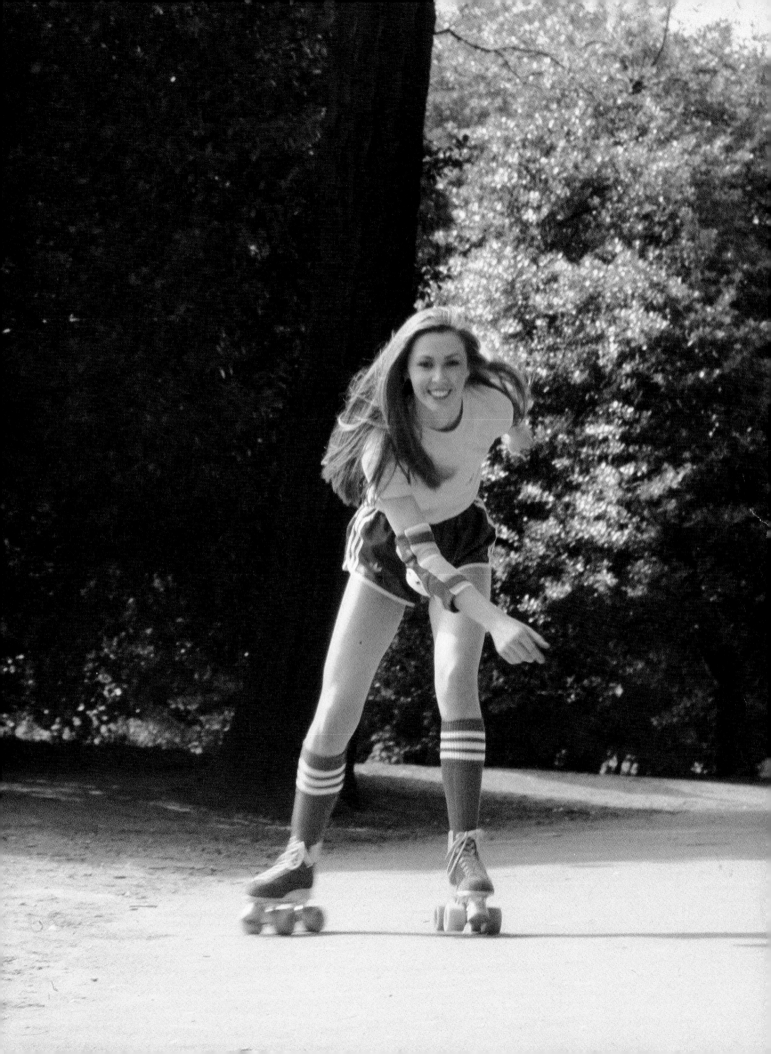

Stamina

Can you cope with heavy exertion? Run without becoming breathless? Does it take a while for you to simmer down again? The real test of fitness is your aerobic capacity. Aerobic means 'with air or oxygen' and the activities which fall into this category include running, brisk walking, cycling etc. To understand their importance you must know how your cardio-respiratory system works. This consists of your lungs, which take oxygen from the air and pass it through your blood to your heart, and your blood vessels, which carry the blood with oxygen and nutrients all over your body. When your heart pounds and you feel you cannot breathe, it is because your system cannot deliver enough oxygen. With activity, you strengthen and enlarge your heart so that it pumps out more blood per beat. Then it doesn't have to work so hard at maintaining your blood circulation, and is therefore under less strain.

To test your stamina, run on the spot, lifting your feet about six inches off the floor; carry on until you feel breathless, but don't strain yourself. If you are under 50 you should be able to keep going for about three minutes quite comfortably. If you feel terrible after one minute, stop immediately. You are not fit. Or try walking briskly up and down a fairly long staircase. If you can do it three times and still be able to talk because you haven't run out of breath, you're probably quite fit.

The pulse test

This is a more accurate method of assessing your fitness, but it is slightly more complicated. First you need to learn to take your own pulse. There are three good places to do this. The first, and most convenient, is on your wrist. Using three fingers, lightly press your wrist at the base of the thumb joint, palm facing upwards. You should feel the light, steady beat of your heart pumping. The second place is the artery just below your jaw, at the side of your throat – press on one side only so you don't shut off the blood supply. The third is the artery near the front of your ear, towards your temple. If you keep mislaying your wrist pulse, try drawing a small cross on your skin as a guide. To take your pulse rate, use the second hand of a clock or watch and count your pulse beats. Rather than count a whole minute, you can count for 30 seconds and multiply by two, 15 seconds and multiply by four or six seconds and add a 0. Your resting pulse rate, when you are calm and sitting down, can vary, but averages 75–80 (women), 82–89 (girls), 72–76 (men) and 80–84 (boys).

To test your fitness, you have to assess your pulse rate after exercising. Run on the spot, or step up and down alternately on to the second step of the stairs or a low stool, bench or chair. Do it for 2 minutes, but stop if you feel any strain. Take your pulse immediately you stop. The six-second count will give you a quicker assessment, which would be more accurate because your pulse rate will drop soon after you stop exercising. To calculate your own particular recommended pulse rating, subtract your age from 200, then subtract a handicap of 40. For example, if you are 32, your pulse rating norm, exercising, would be 128. If your pulse is that, you are fine. If it's much higher, you are not fit. Much lower? You must be very fit. As your fitness improves you should reduce your handicap, first to 30 and then to 20, when calculating your recommended pulse rate.

Your Personal Exercise Programme

Exercise can be used in four different ways. Gentle outdoor activities from a round of golf to a walk in the country are good for rest and relaxation. Isometrics, calisthenics (stretching exercises) and weight-lifting improve muscle-building and contouring. Stretching exercises and yoga help your mobility and suppleness. Aerobics – cycling, jogging, skipping rope – improve your cardiovascular conditioning. In women, this last kind of exercise has been neglected and only recently have we come to realize its importance.

Start your exercise programme slowly and gently until your body becomes more supple. Don't move up to more strenuous levels of activity until you're sure your body is able to take it. Never force yourself. *Always* check with your doctor first if you have been ill, are very overweight, over 40, a heavy smoker, suffer from stress, or have any history of heart or back problems. This applies to any kind of exercise you do – isometrics, for instance, may seem gentle enough, but can be dangerous for those with high blood pressure.

What's the minimum exercise you need? I'm afraid I can't give you an easy way out on three minutes a week. You really need about three half-hour sessions a week for the greatest benefit, although 15 minutes a day would be fine if you did it seven days a week. Always begin with some warm-ups before moving on to aerobics and stretching exercises. As you lose weight and become more fit, add weights, try yoga.

Early morning, last thing at night, during a break in the middle of the day – do your exercises whenever you wish. Don't, however, exercise immediately after a heavy meal; wait

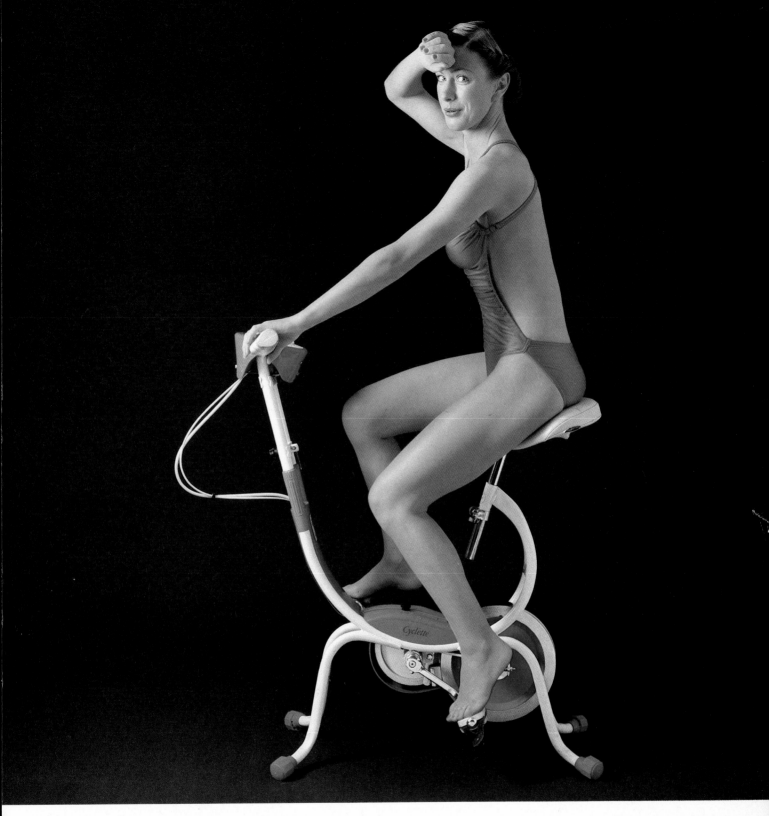

about two hours before beginning. Comfortable, casual clothing is the best kind to wear – preferably a leotard and footless tights. But anything – or nothing – will do so long as it is not tight and constricting. Always wear tennis shoes when running in place. Choose a fairly open space so that you won't feel cramped by furniture. Some of the exercises can be uncomfortable on a bare floor, so if you don't have a carpet, use a rug, blanket or mat.

There are a number of machines on the market that are claimed to help you lose inches and reshape your body. I'm thinking of vibrator belts, electric massagers and machine exercisers. Avoid them. As you know, the only way you can *lose* weight is by dieting, and the best way to tone your body and take up the slack is by exercising your muscles *yourself*. The only 'gadgets' that approximate real exercise are stationary exercise bikes; these can be useful if you prefer to exercise indoors, or live in a city and don't want to fight traffic while you cycle. Most gyms and health clubs have exercise bikes.

Exercise bikes are a good alternative to cycling outdoors – and can be strenuous work!

Posture Pointers

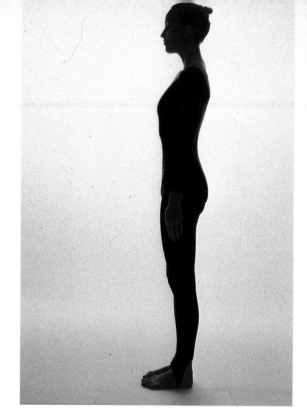

Whether you are fat or thin, the way you carry yourself says a lot about how you feel. Walking, sitting and standing, your body attitudes reveal your moods, energy (or lack of it) and your self-esteem. Above all, good posture can make you appear slimmer whatever your weight, just as bad posture and slumping around can make even slender girls seem thicker. Become aware of your body attitudes and you will improve them.

Body alignment affects your health as well as grace and elegance. Sagging shoulders cramp your chest, stopping you breathing naturally and fully. Slouching cramps your digestive system. Poking your head forward puts strain on your back. Lifting and bending incorrectly leads to back strain and pain.

Standing your ground
Pull yourself up as if an invisible thread were attached from the top of your head to the ceiling, stretching out all your muscles, making you taller. Stand up straight, shoulders back but relaxed and down, not held ramrod stiff or hunched. Hold your chest and ribs high. Pull in your tummy and tuck in your seat, keep your knees together but not stiff, balance your weight evenly on both feet.

Sitting pretty
When you sit down, don't poke your bottom into the chair awkwardly and slump like an old beanbag. Try to descend into the chair as if between two vertical lines. Stand with your back to the chair, the back leg almost touching with the other just in front. Keeping your back straight and your head up, lower yourself into the chair smoothly – as you sink down, your knees bend, moving forward.

Sit deep into the chair, don't slouch. A hard chair is best for long sitting – it gives more support. When you are seated, your back should be straight, tummy tucked in, the weight supported on your sitting bones, not your thighs. Keep your chin and chest high, midriff lifted. Keep legs together, too. Splayed-out legs look ungainly. Don't twine legs together either – crossing your legs can impede circulation so it's a particularly bad idea if you have varicose veins.

Walking gracefully
Pull yourself up straight, without being stiff. Pull in your stomach and seat and do not lead with your chin – keep the top of your head aligned to your body as in standing. Walk relaxed with toes pointing forwards, swinging

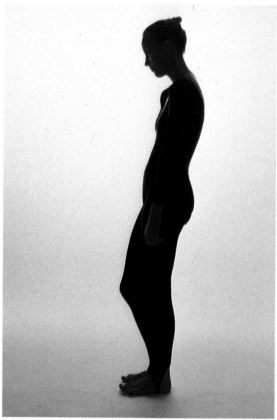

each leg from the hip – not the knee. Traditionally, models trained to walk more gracefully by practising with a large book balanced on their heads – the body had to be aligned properly for it to stay there unaided.

Bending and lifting
Backache is one of the commonest pains of all and may be caused by lifting heavy objects incorrectly or by bending awkwardly. Do not

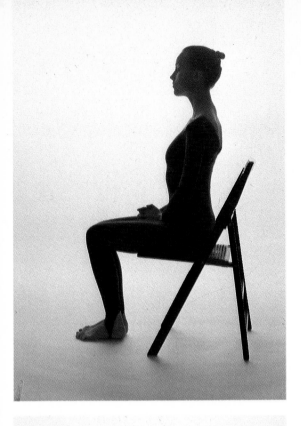

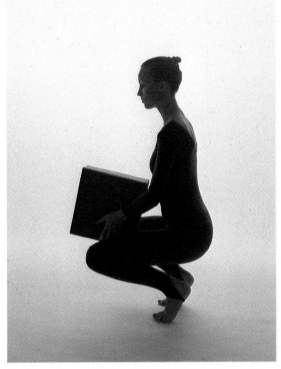

The top row shows the correct way to stand, sit, and bend to lift things; the bottom row shows the incorrect way. Notice how big a difference posture makes to the way you appear to the world: standing properly, you look at ease, in control, ready for anything; slumping, you look worried, tired, too beaten to cope with anything.

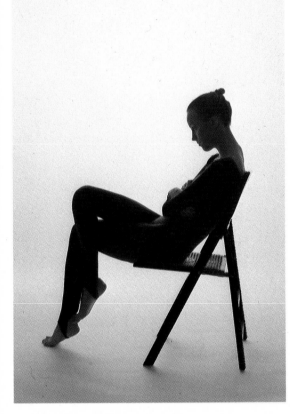

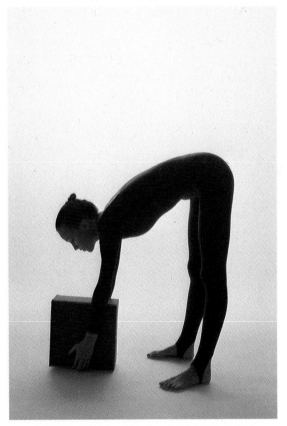

bend forwards to pick something up, taking the strain on your back and shoulders. Instead, bend your knees and take the strain on your thigh muscles. Always find ways to take the strain *off* your back and use the muscles in your legs, arms and stomach – which benefit from the exercise.

When shopping, distribute the weight between two bags instead of one. When stooping, do not bend down from the waist with feet together, but bend your knees, with one foot forward bearing your weight, arm back for balance. When carrying a suitcase or heavy bag, change hands frequently to distribute the load. Do not slump to one side with shoulder dragged down, weight on one hip, neck craned with the strain. Instead, balance your body weight, keeping your back straight, arms and shoulders level, tummy and seat muscles pulled in, and head up to straighten your spine.

43

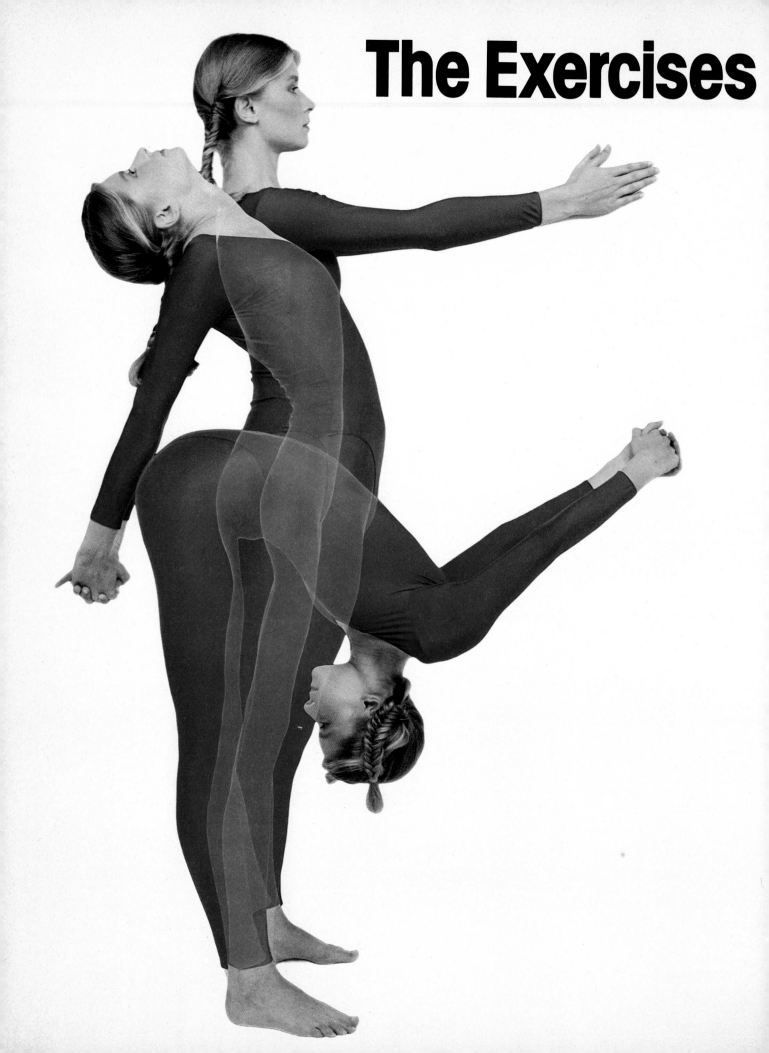

The Exercises

WARM UPS

Warm up your body before embarking on any vigorous exercise session. Even if it is only for three or four minutes, you will prepare your muscles, make your joints more flexible, and improve your suppleness. Pick two or three from these examples and build them into your programme.

Stretch ups
Stand up straight, legs together, arms at your sides. Rise on your toes and swing your arms up and over your head, touching hands. Stretch your body up, pulling in your seat and stomach. Return to first position. Repeat about 10–15 times.

Side benders
Stand with feet apart, arms at your sides, head straight. Lean sideways, sliding one hand down the side of your leg. Straighten up again, then lean to the other side. Repeat 10 times.

Shoulder rolls
Stand, feet apart, arms at your sides. Shrug your shoulders up to your ears, then bring them back and down and reverse the action, making a rolling movement. Do 5–10 times.

Penguin flaps
Stand with feet slightly apart, arms at your sides. Stretch out your arms sideways, letting wrists go limp, and flap your arms up and down at your sides quite briskly while counting to 10.

Forward flops
Stand with feet together, arms at your sides. Drop forward from the waist, like a rag doll, keeping your arms and shoulders relaxed. Keep legs straight but not tense. Straighten up slowly. Repeat 3–5 times.

Knee pulls
Stand, feet together, arms at your sides. Raise one knee as high as you can, grasp it with both hands and pull it towards your body. Keep your back and head straight. Repeat with other leg. Do 10 times.

Hip circles
Stand with feet slightly apart, hands on your hips. Pull in your stomach, then rotate your pelvis, as if using a hula-hoop, first one way, then the other. Repeat about 10 times.

Leg stretchers
Face a wall, tree or heavy stationary object. Place your hands flat against it at shoulder level, with arms outstretched, and slowly shuffle backwards. Keep your feet flat on the ground. Go sufficiently far back so you feel the strain on the backs of your knees and legs. Hold for about 20 seconds. Go back to stage one and repeat 2–3 times.

Leg swings
Stand straight with one arm resting on the back of a chair for support, and swing one leg forwards and backwards. Turn to face the other direction and swing the other leg. Repeat 10–15 times.

Stretch ups ▶

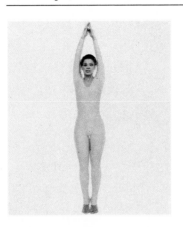

Side benders ▶

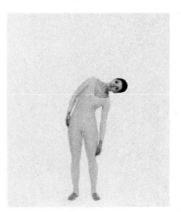

Shoulder rolls ▶

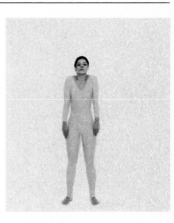

Penguin flaps ▶

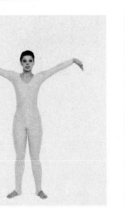

Forward flops ▶

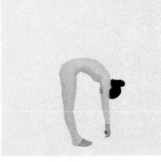

Knee pulls ▶

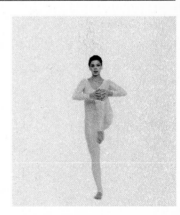

Hip circles ▶

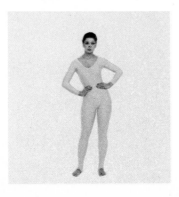

Leg stretchers ▶

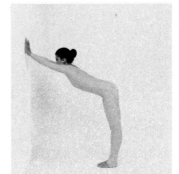

Leg swings ▶

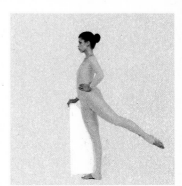

THE FITNESS PROGRAMMES

The exercises that follow have been graded A, B and C. For easy reference, they carry colour codes: A, for the easiest exercises, is yellow; B, for those of intermediate level, is blue; C, for the advanced exercises, is red. These pages give ideas for complete exercise programmes for each of these levels; pages 52–59 suggest exercises to help tone specific parts of your body. Many of the exercises can be adapted to be more or less difficult; for instance, a leg-raising exercise will be much harder if you do it very slowly. Before you begin, determine which category suits you best. You should have a good idea of your fitness if you did the tests in the previous section. If you want more guidance, answer the following questions. If you get more C's than anything else you can probably do a more active programme. B's? A moderate programme. A's? A gentle programme.

- Are you   A Very overweight   B A bit overweight   C Normal weight
- How old are you?   A Over 50   B 30's–40   C Teens–20's
- Do you smoke?   A Yes – quite a lot or a great deal   B A little   C No
- Did your parents   A Both die from heart disease?   B Did one die early from heart disease?   C Did they live to a ripe old age or are they still alive and healthy?
- How do you rate your personality?   A Tense, aggressive, frustrated, irritable?   B An up and down personality, sometimes tense, sometimes relaxed?   C Easy-going, confident, content?
- Have you done any exercises before?   A Never   B Infrequently   C Frequently
- What type of work do you do?   A Sedentary, sitting down most of the time   B Fairly active   C Very active
- How is your health?   A Not good   B Fairly good   C Very good

Fitness Programme A

This is a very gentle exercise regime which includes aerobics and movements to help your suppleness and strength. Follow it if you are overweight, smoke, have a sedentary job, are not used to exercise.

Running on the spot
Run in place lightly on your toes, raising your feet a few inches from the floor. Begin by running for half a minute. Gradually build up your endurance, lifting your legs higher and running for longer as you grow stronger. This exercise will help improve the efficiency of your heart and lungs.

Arm circles
Stand up straight with feet apart, head up, tummy and seat tucked in, arms outstretched to shoulder height. With palms up, rotate your arms backwards 12 times in circles, beginning with small circles and increasing to larger ones. Relax. Repeat in the other direction. Do several times to improve your suppleness.

Legs away
Lie on your back on the floor with your arms at your sides, legs together. Slowly draw your knees up towards your chest, bringing your heels as close to your buttocks as you can. Keep knees and feet together. Slowly stretch your legs straight to point at the ceiling, then just as slowly bring them back to the knees-bent position. Straighten out. Do this about 3 times to start with and gradually increase over 4 weeks. This is particularly good for your stomach.

Wall press offs
Stand at arms' length from a wall, with your legs and arms straight, hands pointing upwards on the wall. Bending your elbows, lean towards the wall until your chest touches it. Straighten up your arms to return to standing position. Repeat 8 times. This is a good strengthening exercise.

Waist bends
Stand up straight, arms at your sides, feet apart, legs straight. Raise your right arm over your head and lean over to the left, chest high, seat and stomach tucked in, arm stretching over your head towards the left. Feel the pull. Hold for a count of 4, then stand up straight again. Repeat with your left arm. Begin with 4 of these and increase to 12.

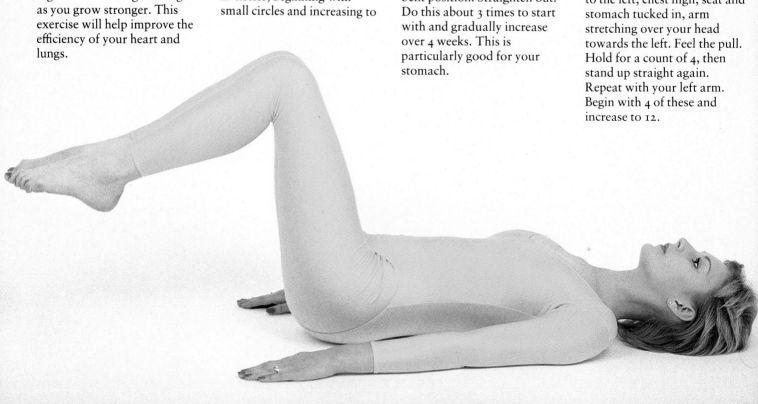

Running on the spot ▶   **Arm circles ▶**

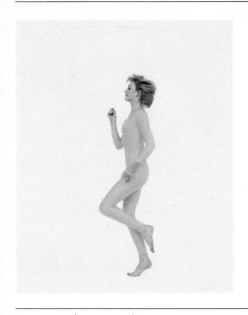 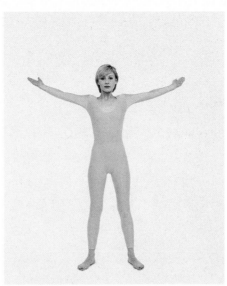 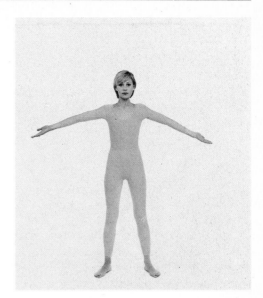

Legs away ▶   **Wall press offs ▶**

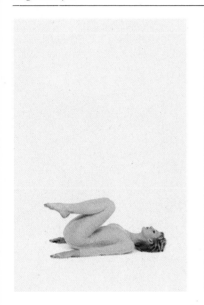 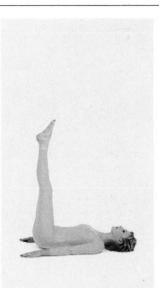 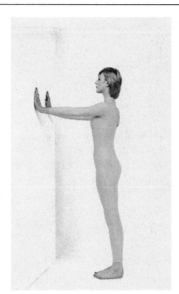 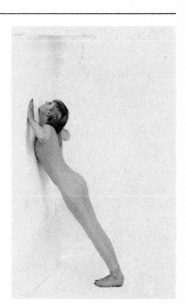

Waist bends ▶

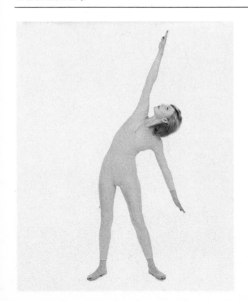 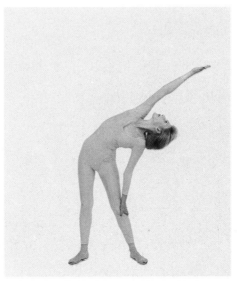 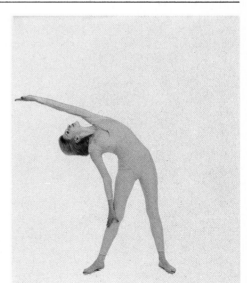

Fitness Programme B

This intermediate group of exercises is designed for those who are a bit overweight, not too fit, perhaps over 30. It is also the next stage for those who have begun with programme A and now feel supple enough to move on. If you start here and really feel the strain, don't pursue it. Instead, work through the A exercises until you are in better shape.

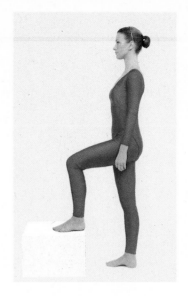
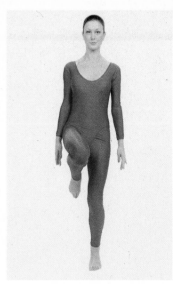

Step exercise
To do this, use the stairs, a sturdy low box or a stool. Move forwards and backwards from floor to step or stool as follows: left foot up, right foot up, left foot down, right foot down. Take it slowly to begin with and increase your speed over time.

Run and stride jumps
Stand with feet together, arms at your sides. Run on the spot, raising your feet at least 4–5 inches off the floor. Each time your right foot touches the floor count 1. After 50 runs, do 10 stride jumps – with feet together and arms at your sides, jump so your feet are about 18 inches apart when you land. At the same time, raise your arms to shoulder level. Jump again so your feet are together, arms at your sides when you land. Do about 100 runs, with stride jumps twice.

Shoulder push
Another good strengthening exercise. Place your hands about shoulder width apart on the edge of a heavy chair or a bed and move your feet backwards until your back and legs are in a straight line. Your arms should be straight, your weight supported on your hands and the balls of your feet. Bend at the elbows and lower your body until your chest touches the edge. Push up, straightening your arms. Do this several times.

Knee push ups
Lie face down on the floor, legs together and knees straight, with your palms on the floor under your shoulders and your elbows bent.

Straighten your arms to push your body off the floor, but only from your knees. Start with 8 and work up to 20. This is an excellent exercise for improving your strength.

Twist and bend
Lie on the floor with your legs straight, arms stretched sideways at shoulder level. First bend your right knee towards your chest, then your left knee. Drop both knees to the right, together; then, swinging over, drop them to the left. Bring both knees up to your chest again. Stretch out as first position. Repeat 18–25 times (under 30) or 10–15 times (over 30). Very good for your stomach.

Crouch jumps
Stand with your feet slightly apart, arms at your sides. Bend your knees to a crouching position, then spring up lightly, jumping up in the air as high as you feel you can manage. Begin with 5–10 (under 30) or 4–8 (over 30) and build up as you feel able. Good for legs and thighs.

Stretch and clap
Stand up straight, feet wide apart, hands by your sides. Bend your right knee, stretch out your left leg and stretch your arms to the right, clapping above your right shoulder. Then bend down to the left, stretching your right leg, bending your left knee, and clap your hands near your left foot. Stretch up again and clap your hands above your right shoulder. Face front and repeat on the other side. A good stretching exercise, do this 15–20 times (under 30) or 10–15 times (over 30).

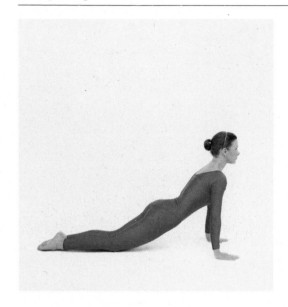

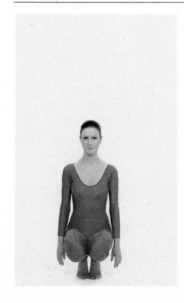
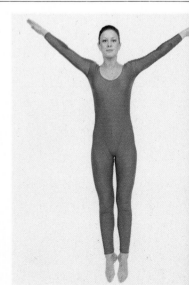

Shoulder push ▶

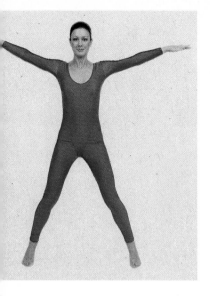 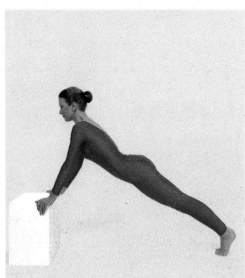 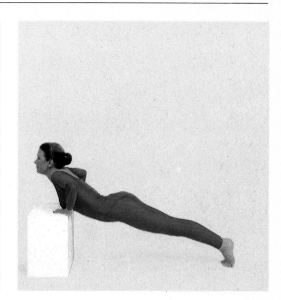

Twist and bend ▶

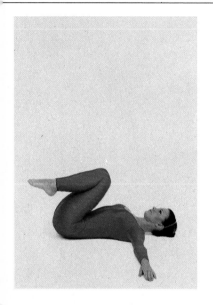 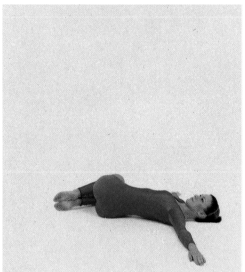 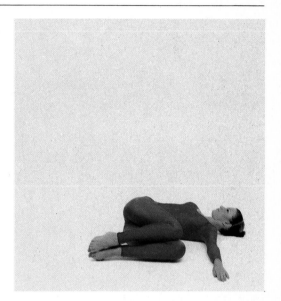

Stretch and clap ▶

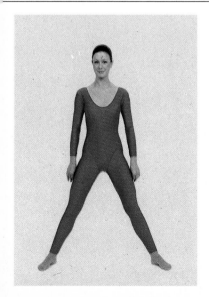 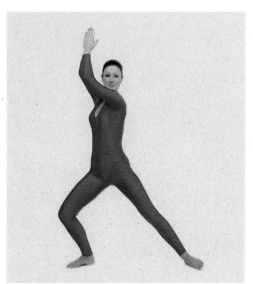 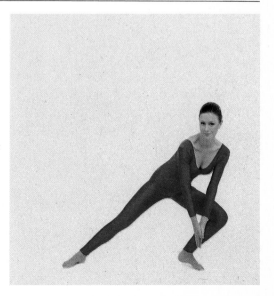

Fitness Programme C

You should be extremely fit and supple by the time you do this series of exercises. To make the exercises stretch you even more, take the appropriate ones more slowly. Raised leg ups and The flyer, for instance, can be made more difficult by going more slowly still, and by holding each final position to a count of 10 or more.

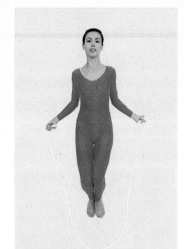

Skipping

Stand straight with your feet together, holding a skipping rope behind them. Bring the rope up over your head as you rise to your toes, then jump with your feet together and pass the rope underneath. Repeat, trying to maintain an even rhythm. Don't be flat-footed – always jump on the balls of your feet. A less strenuous method is to hop on one foot only, alternating feet. If you're under 30, skip for 1 minute to begin with and work up to 4 minutes. Over 30, start with 30 seconds and work up to 2 minutes.

Squat thrusts

Stand with your arms at your sides and feet slightly apart. Bend your knees to a squat position, balancing on the balls of your feet, and place your hands on the floor to the sides of your knees. Thrust your feet backwards to a push-up position, legs straight and toes on the floor. Spring back to the squat position. Do a set of 5 before standing up.

The flyer

Lie face down with your legs together and straight, arms stretched out sideways to shoulder level. Raise your head, upper body and arms off the floor as high as you can, at the same time raising your legs, but keeping your knees straight. Relax. Repeat 15 times (under 30) or 8 times (over 30).

Sit ups

Lie on your back, legs straight, elbows bent with your hands beneath your head. Without moving from your hips down, slowly raise the top half of your body into a sitting position, then lean forward and touch your right elbow to your left knee. Slowly go back to the first position. Repeat, this time touching your left elbow to your right knee. If your feet have a tendency to move, secure them under a suitable piece of furniture to keep them stationary. Do 15–20 times (under 30) or 10–15 (over 30).

Arm flings

Stand up straight, feet slightly apart, upper arms extended at shoulder level. Bend your elbows so your fingers almost touch in front of your chest, then press your elbows backwards and upwards. Return to second position, then fling your arms out, back and up as far as you can. Return to first position. Do the complete exercise 20 times (under 30) and 12 times (over 30). Work up to 30 and 22 times as you become more fit.

Raised leg ups

Sit on the floor and lean back on your hands, legs straight and together, toes pointed. Raise your buttocks off the floor with your hands providing support, until your torso and legs make a straight line – only feet and hands touching the floor. Raise your right leg slowly, still keeping your body straight and the toes pointed. Lift the leg as high as you can, keeping the knee straight, then lower. Repeat with left leg. Do 10 and work up to 16 (under 30) or 6 and work up to 12 (over 30). This is good for your waist and torso.

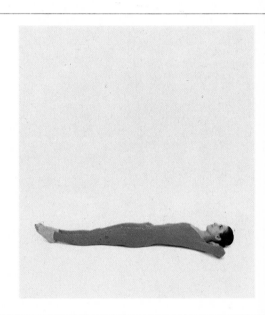

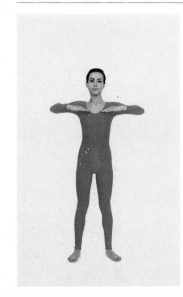

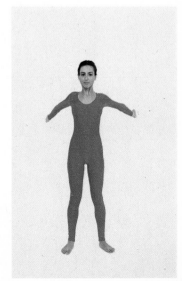

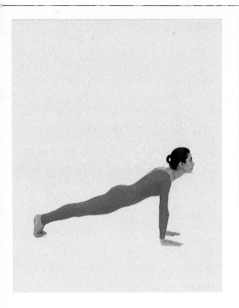
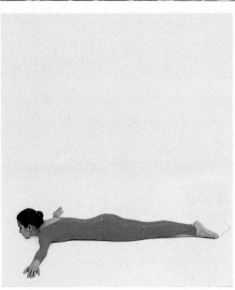
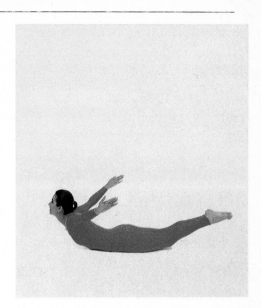

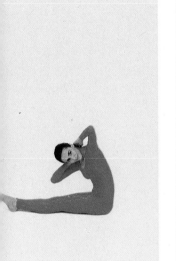
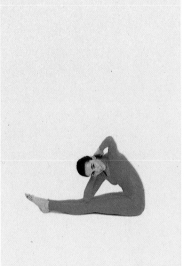
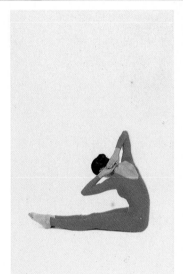
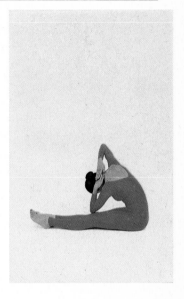

Raised leg ups ▶

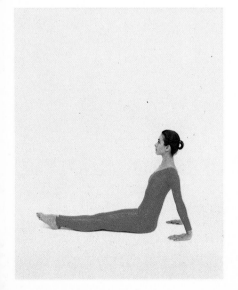
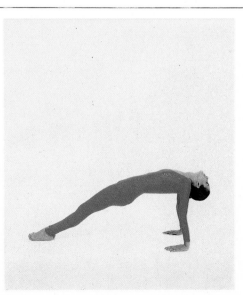
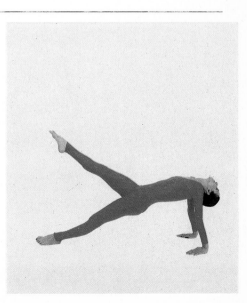

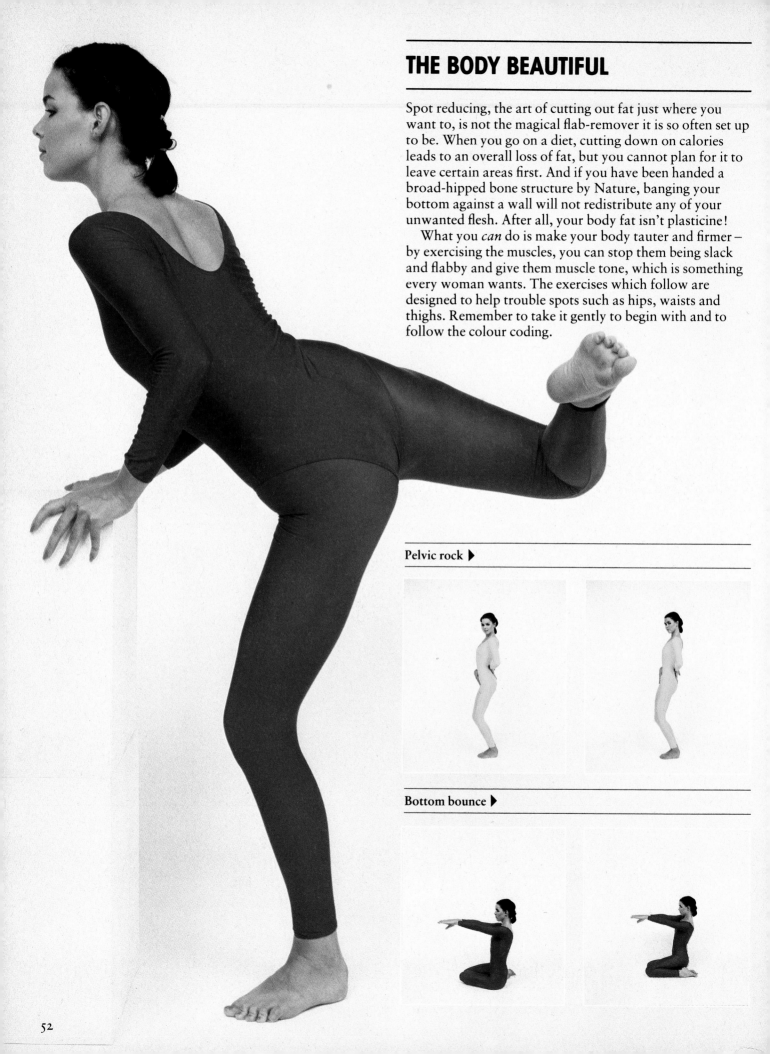

THE BODY BEAUTIFUL

Spot reducing, the art of cutting out fat just where you want to, is not the magical flab-remover it is so often set up to be. When you go on a diet, cutting down on calories leads to an overall loss of fat, but you cannot plan for it to leave certain areas first. And if you have been handed a broad-hipped bone structure by Nature, banging your bottom against a wall will not redistribute any of your unwanted flesh. After all, your body fat isn't plasticine!

What you *can* do is make your body tauter and firmer – by exercising the muscles, you can stop them being slack and flabby and give them muscle tone, which is something every woman wants. The exercises which follow are designed to help trouble spots such as hips, waists and thighs. Remember to take it gently to begin with and to follow the colour coding.

Pelvic rock ▶

Bottom bounce ▶

Your Bottom Half

Heavy thighs, wide bottoms and fleshy hips are problems shared by many women. Your bottom is the part of your body that seems to get the least exercise. Big thighs often seem to remain even after a significant weight loss. Exercise can firm all this flesh, but you must work hard at it. Be consistent, and don't expect results too soon. All exercises are illustrated unless marked with an asterisk at the end.

Seat walk

For buttocks. Sit on the floor, legs outstretched, hands off the floor and pointing straight towards your toes. 'Walk' on your buttocks, inching your way right across the room, lifting your hip off the floor and reaching forward with one leg at a time. Once you've wriggled your way to one side of the room, wriggle backwards in reverse gear.*

Pelvic rock

For buttocks. Stand with your feet together. Bend your knees a little and place the palm of your right hand on your stomach and the back of your left hand on your buttocks. Push your bottom out to a count of 2 and tuck it in and push your hips forward to a count of 2. Repeat 10 times.

Cycling

For hips. Lie flat on your back, arms outstretched at sides, legs straight and together. Lift legs up towards the ceiling and pretend you're riding a bike, cycling in the air. Begin with about 25 cycles, and work up to more.*

The Slide

For thighs. Stand up straight with your back against a wall, feet together and arms at sides. *Slowly* slide down the wall until you are squatting on the balls of your feet, with your knees bent. Keep your back straight and hold for a count of 10. Repeat 4 times. This really pulls, so work up to it gradually, then increase the length of time you hold the position.

Bottom bounce

For buttocks. Sit on the floor, leaning on your left hip with your legs bent over to the right under you. Stretch out your arms in front, keeping your back straight, and pull in your stomach. Still keeping your arms out and your back straight, twist your hips to the right side. Then twist them back to the left again. Keep your legs together throughout. Repeat about 6 times.

Scissor snips

For hips. Lie on your right side with your upper right arm extended and your right hand supporting your head, your left hand on the floor in front and your legs straight and together. Keeping your body still, raise your left leg straight and as high as you can. Lower your leg and repeat 8 times, then turn around and repeat with the other leg.

Kick back

For buttocks. Kneel on all fours, with hands and knees about 8 inches apart, keeping your arms and thighs at right angles to your torso. Kick your right leg up and back as high as you can, then lower it, bend the knee and bring the leg up to your chest, bending your head down to meet it. Go into the all-fours position again, and repeat with the other leg. Do this with each leg about 8 times.

Lift off

For buttocks. Push a chair near a wall for support and hold on to the back. Bend your legs and lean on the left leg as you lift the right leg behind you as high as you can. Straighten out your knees, then bend them again, still keeping the right leg high. Repeat last 2 positions 4 times, then repeat with other leg.

Scissor snips ▶

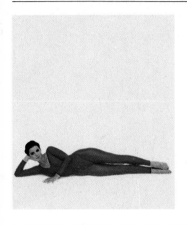 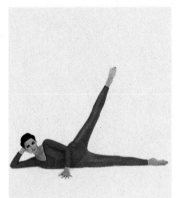

Kick back ▶

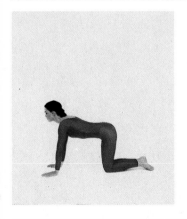 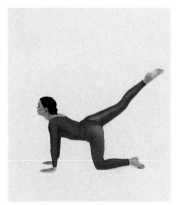 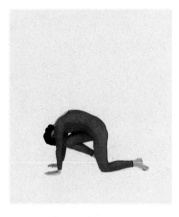

Lift off ▶

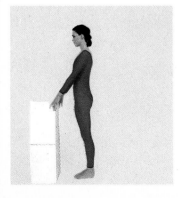 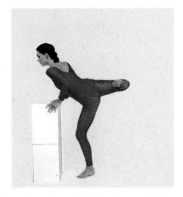 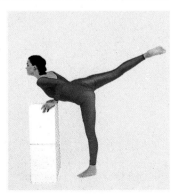

The body bow ▶

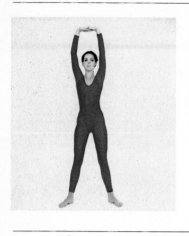
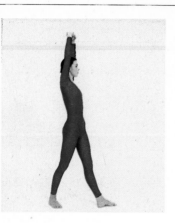
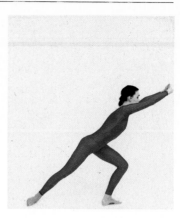

The body bow
For hips. Stand with your feet apart, arms stretched over your head, fingers interlinked. Twist your whole body around to the left. Then, keeping your feet the same distance apart, change the direction of your feet so that your left one faces straight ahead, your right one points diagonally outwards. Slowly sway your body forward, bending your left knee hard and keeping your right leg and back straight. Return to the

Leg crook ▶   The jerk ▶

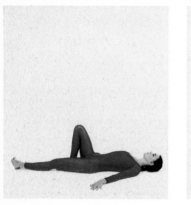
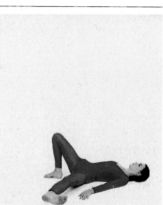
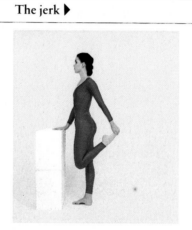
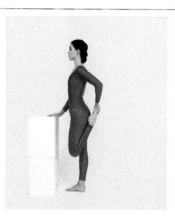

Scissors stretch ▶   The slant ▶

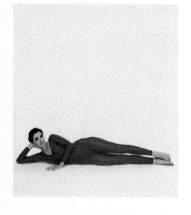
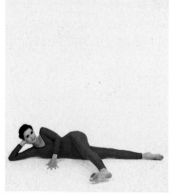
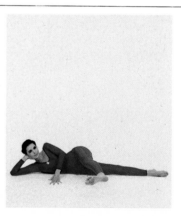
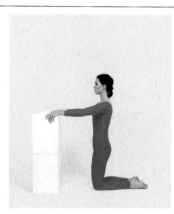

Circles in the air ▶   Cross overs ▶

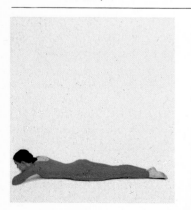
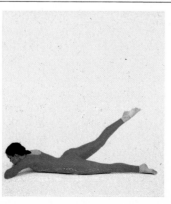
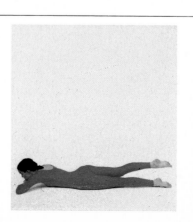
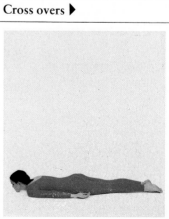

first position and repeat, this time twisting to the right and bending your right knee. Repeat 5 times.

Knee bends

For buttocks and thighs. Stand with your feet together, arms outstretched in front at shoulder level, palms down. Breathing in, rise up on to the balls of your feet, stretching up and tightening your buttocks. Keeping your back straight, bend your knees and breathe out as you slowly

lower yourself to a squatting position. Repeat 5 times.*

Leg kicks

A good all-over leg exercise. Use a table for support, high enough so you can kick under it. Stand near it with your feet together, stomach tucked in, back straight, one hand touching. Keeping your legs straight, swing your right leg up and back, then out to the side and across the left leg towards the table. Repeat 6 times with each leg.*

The Z exercise ▶

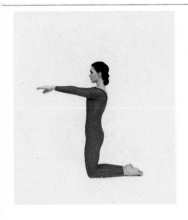
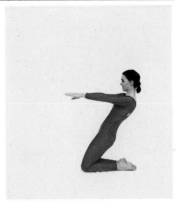

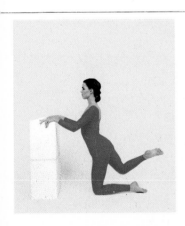
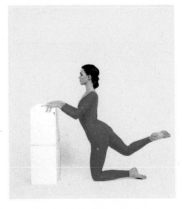

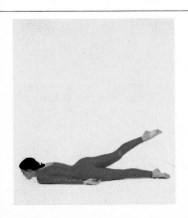
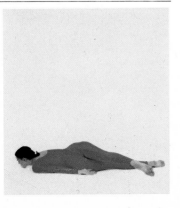

Bottom lift

For buttocks. Lie on your back with your knees bent, arms outstretched at sides. Tense your buttock muscles and lift them high off the ground, raising your heels up. Hold the position and raise and lower your heels 10 times. Relax and repeat 5 times.*

Leg crook

For hips. Lie on the floor with one leg straight, the other bent with your foot flat on the floor. Press the middle of your back into the floor, pull in your stomach, tuck in your seat and pull up your pelvic-floor muscles. Now swing the straight leg out sideways and back, keeping it just off the ground. Be sure your knee is still straight and your foot turned up. Repeat with the other leg, then repeat 5 times.

The jerk

For hips. Face the back of a chair and hold the side of it with your right hand, standing with your legs straight. With your left hand, catch hold of your left foot. Keeping the rest of your body straight, pull the left leg towards you. Repeat 5 times with each leg.

The Z exercise

For thighs. Kneel on the floor with your back straight. Raise your arms straight out in front at shoulder level. Keeping your body straight, lean back slowly as far as you can without hurting yourself or losing your balance. Your hips will be forward, shoulders back. Repeat 5 times.

Thigh press

For thighs. Stand by a table or chest of drawers to support yourself with one hand. With your feet apart, put your weight on the outside leg, at the same time bending your elbow and slightly lowering your head towards the support. Push hard on your feet and pull away from the support with your hips, keeping your legs straight. Draw your inner thighs together without moving your feet. Relax. Repeat 3 times on each side.*

Scissors stretch

For thighs. Lie on your right side, leaning on your elbow and supporting yourself with your hands. Stretch your legs out straight. Bring your straight left leg over so that it lies at a right angle to your body. Flex your foot and lift and lower your left leg, keeping it at the 90° angle. You will be able to feel a pull. Change sides, then repeat about 10 times.

The slant

For buttocks. This is one of the exercises devised by the expert Lotte Berk. Kneel on the floor and hold on to the edge of a table for support. With your weight on your left knee, raise and extend your right leg diagonally behind you with the knee slightly bent, then incline backwards over the extended leg. Without moving your body, roll your right hip forwards – this is difficult and may take a lot of practice. Finally, raise and lower the right leg 5 times. If you are doing the exercise correctly, you will only be able to raise your leg a few inches. Repeat with other leg.

Circles in the air

For hips. Lie on your stomach on the floor, resting your chin on your arms. Raise your right leg, keeping the knee straight and, moving your leg clockwise, try to draw a large circle in the air. Lower and repeat with your left leg. Now lift the right leg and draw a counter-clockwise circle, then repeat with left leg. Work up to 6 circles each way with each leg.

Cross overs

For thighs. Lie face down on the floor, arms by your sides, chin touching the floor. Raise your right leg as high as you can, keeping it straight, and move it across the left leg to touch the floor on the other side. Raise the leg high in the air again, without bending the knee, and touch the floor on the right side. Repeat with your left leg. Do this about 8 times with each leg.

Your Top Half

Your stomach is an area of the body where exercise can yield particularly good results, for although the muscles can go slack even when you are not very fat, they can also be toned to flatness with a bit of effort. Waists should nip in to accentuate your feminine curves; every waist looks better with good posture and you will have a better body line if you exercise consistently. Unless you play a sport regularly, your arms can grow slack and flabby; always try to include at least one arm exercise in your programme to keep the muscles toned. When you do bust exercises, you are really toning the platform of muscles attached to the breast wall called the pectorals. The breasts themselves are mammary glands sunk in connective tissue and fat, surrounded by envelopes of skin which give them shape; they contain no muscle. Exercising the pectorals, however, will help uplift. Exercises marked * are not illustrated.

The hook
For stomach. Lie on your back with your legs straight, arms at your sides. Bend your right knee and bring it to your chest, keeping the left leg straight. Lower and straighten the right leg slowly. Repeat with your left leg, and then repeat 10 times.*

Chair raises
For stomach. Sit on the edge of a hard chair. Lean against the back of the chair with your legs extended straight out, feet on the ground. Raise your right leg high and stretch out to touch it with your left hand. Relax. Repeat with the other leg, then repeat 5 times.*

Swing it
For waist. Stand with your feet apart, arms outstretched at sides to shoulder level. Keeping your arms straight, swing them forwards and backwards, twisting your waist. Keep legs steady. Repeat several times.

Waist circles
For waist. Stand with your feet apart, clasp your hands above your head and raise your head to look at your fingers. Now swing your arms, head and upper torso in circles, bending to the side, dropping down to the floor, up towards the other side, then back so that your arms are above your head again. Keep your legs straight throughout. Do this first in one direction, then the other, about 5 times.*

Windmills
For arms and shoulders. Stand with your feet apart, arms at sides. Make large backwards circles with your arms, moving them one after the other or both at once, whichever is more comfortable. Repeat 10 times.

Arm lift
For arms. Sit on the edge of a chair, gripping the seat with your hands. Push on your hands, with your arms straight, and lift yourself off the seat, legs straight out in front of you, keeping feet flat on the floor. Keep your back straight. Relax and repeat 8 times.

Arm shrugs
For arms. Sit on the floor with your legs crossed and back straight. Stretch out your arms, palms up. Draw your elbows in towards your waist, then shrug your arms forwards and backwards. Repeat 20 times.

Swing it ▶

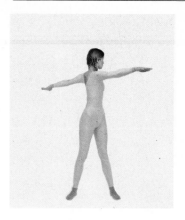
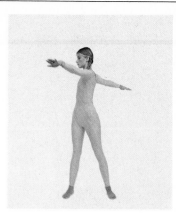

Arm lift ▶

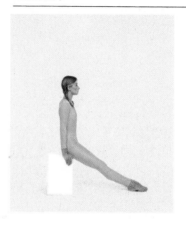
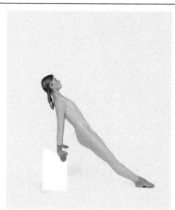

Elbow arcs ▶

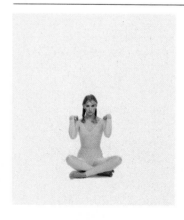
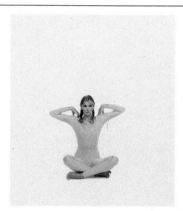

The metronome ▶

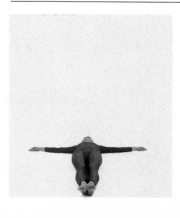
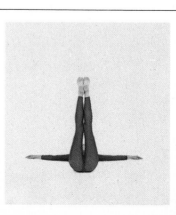

Windmills ▶

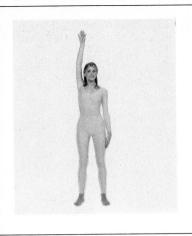 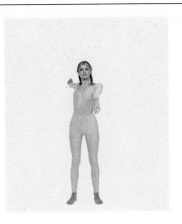 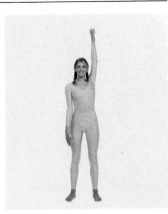

Arm shrugs ▶

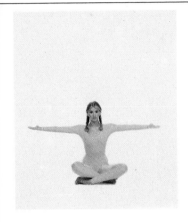 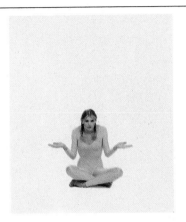 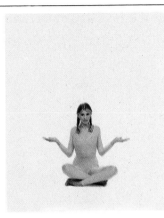

Wrist grips ▶　　　Close up ▶

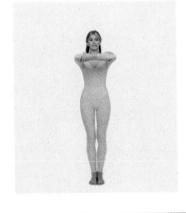 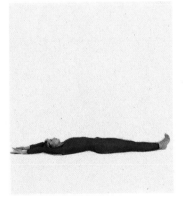 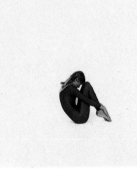

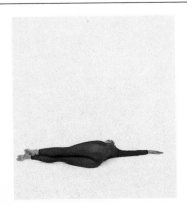 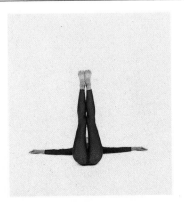 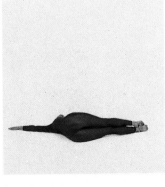

Elbow arcs

For bust. Sit cross-legged on the floor and put your fingertips on your shoulders. Describe circles in the air with your elbows. Do 10 times. If you wish, do this first with one arm, then the other.

Wrist grips

For bust. Stand up straight and stretch out your arms in front of you at shoulder level. Bend your elbows and grasp your wrists firmly so that your forearms, upper arms and shoulders form a rough square. Grip your wrists tightly and force your hands to slide up your forearms to your elbows. Do this 20 times a day for several months if you want results.

Wall games.

For bust. Stand with your back against a wall, legs straight, arms stretched up straight in the air over your head. Press your arms back against the wall, pushing your chest and stomach forward. Relax, then repeat 5 times.*

Close up

For stomach. Lie flat on your back on the floor with your arms out straight behind your head. Sit up and swing your arms forward as you bring your knees up to your chest. Keep your arms stiff and your toes pointed; your hands should touch your toes in the final position. Repeat three times.

The metronome

For stomach. Lie on your back on the floor with your knees straight, arms outstretched. Lift your legs up together until they are at right angles to your body. Then, bending at the hips, push the small of your back into the floor and lower your legs slowly over to the right, lift them, and take them over to the left. Swing legs from side to side about 8 times, keeping them straight throughout.

Tummy toner

For stomach. This is another Lotte Berk exercise. Lie on your back, bending your knees so that your feet are flat on the floor and your heels are close to your bottom. Stretch your arms out behind your head. Push your spine against the floor so that it lies flat and, without moving your lower back, raise your head and shoulders off the floor, stretching your arms up and together as you do so. Hold for 5 seconds, relax and repeat.*

Elbow twists

For waist. Sit on the floor with legs straight and wide apart, back straight and hands clasped behind your head. Twist and bend your body so that your right elbow touches your left knee. Return to straight position. Now twist and bend so that your left elbow touches your right knee. Keep your legs as straight as possible throughout. Repeat 8 times.

Curl ups

For waist. Lie on your back on the floor with your knees bent and your feet and lower legs resting on the seat of a firm chair. Interlock your hands behind your head. Tuck your chin into your chest and slowly curl your body forward into a sitting position, then return to the floor. Do 5 times. An alternative is to stretch your arms out behind your head when you are lying down, then swing yourself forward so your head is over your knees. Too difficult? Try grasping your legs just below the knees to help you get up.

Book lifts

For bust. Lie on your back holding a heavy book in each hand. Extend your arms behind your head, keeping your legs and arms straight and toes pointed. Pull in your tummy and keep your body stretched taut. Lift the books over your head, straight up so your arms are at right angles to your body. Hold for a count of 4. Repeat 5 times.*

Elbow twists ▶

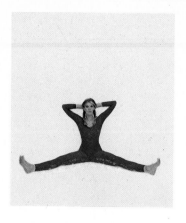 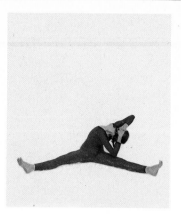 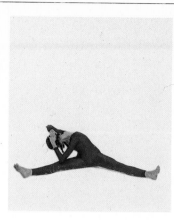

Chest expander ▶

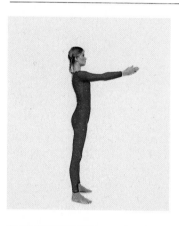 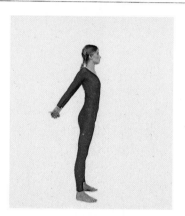 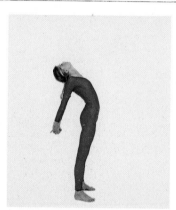

Leg ups ▶

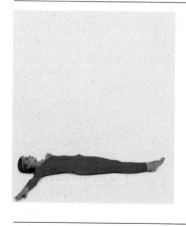 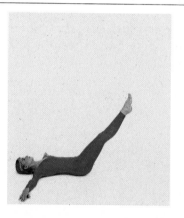 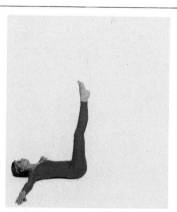

Chair lifts ▶

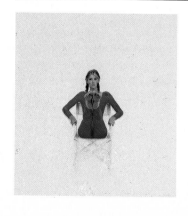 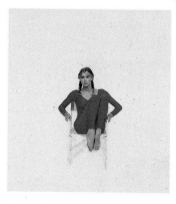 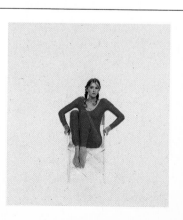

Curl ups ▶

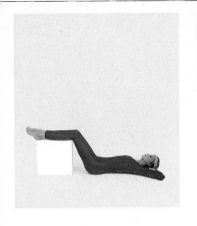
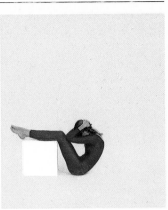

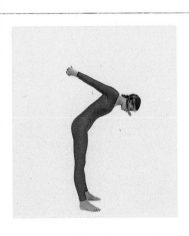
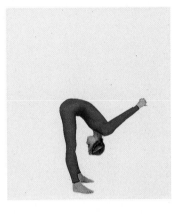

Hand slides ▶

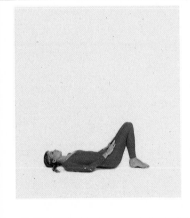
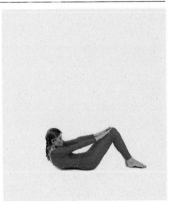

Jack knife ▶

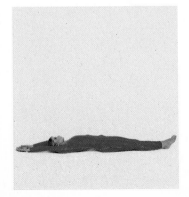
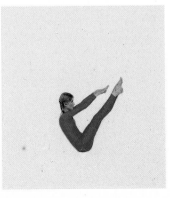

Wall fall

For bust. Stand straight, an arm's length away from a wall. Place your hands on the wall, palms facing inwards, fingers pointing towards each other but hardly touching. Keeping your body straight, slowly bend your elbows, pressing on your palms, and lean forward until your forehead touches the wall. Do not bend at the waist; the line of your body should be unbroken. Hold for about 10 seconds, then slowly return to the standing position, pushing with your palms. Do 3 times.

Chest expander

For bust. Stand up straight, your feet slightly apart, arms stretched forward, palms together. In a wide circling motion, keeping arms straight, bring your arms behind your back and clap your hands together. Slowly bend backwards, looking up. Lean back as far as you can. Now bend forward, hands still clasped together, and bring your arms up over your back. Bend at the waist, with your head hanging down, elbows straight. Hold for 10 seconds. Straighten up slowly, relax, and repeat once.

Leg ups

For stomach. This exercise is based on the yoga position, The Pump. Lie on your back on the floor with your arms extended, palms down. With your legs together and straight, slowly raise them, taking about 10–15 seconds to bring them to a vertical position. By taking your time, you make the exercise more demanding and therefore better for tightening your

muscles. Hold this position for 5 seconds, then lower both legs slowly to the floor. Repeat 6 times.

Hand slides

For stomach. This is another exercise based on yoga. Lie on your back on the floor, with your knees bent so that your feet are flat to the floor. Place your hands on your thighs and, slowly lifting your head, raise your upper body off the floor, sliding your hands up your thighs so your fingertips are almost touching your kneecaps. Don't slide too far, or the exercise becomes easy. Keep your back as straight as you can and hold the position for at least 5 seconds. Slowly lower to the floor, relax, and repeat 3–4 times.

Chair lifts

For waist. Sit in a chair, holding on to the arms. Balancing on your hips by pushing down on your arms, lift your feet off the ground and bend your knees towards your chin. Straighten your legs in front, then bend your knees towards your left shoulder, pointing your feet to the right. Bend knees towards right shoulder, pointing your feet to the left. Bend knees towards your chin and move them from side to side in a fan-like movement. Repeat 5 times.

Jack knife

For waist. Lie flat on the floor, legs together, arms outstretched above your head. Quickly bring your legs and arms up at the same time, keeping them straight, and lift your head in an attempt to touch your toes. Do 5 times.

Isometrics

Isometrics are another good way of exercising your 'top half' – and can also tone other parts of your body that may not get much attention, such as the insides of your thighs. They are take-it-easy exercises which contract muscles instead of expanding them. To tone your breasts, try lifting your elbows, clasping your hands together and pressing your palms hard against each other. A good isometric exercise for your arms is to stand in an open doorway, press the outsides of your fists against the doorposts at shoulder height, and try to force the doorway apart with your fists. If you have high blood pressure or heart problems, check with your doctor before doing any isometrics.

Working with Weights

The recent increase in body consciousness has led many women to take up sports and do aerobic exercises to improve their stamina and to attend exercise and dance classes to make themselves more supple. Strength has largely been ignored, but without strength *and* endurance, you cannot do any exercise properly, or live your life as enthusiastically and healthily as you'd like.

For the modern women of today, the new word to think about is *muscles*! No, I don't mean you should train to have the biceps of a Mr Universe. Muscular fitness simply helps to stop sagging stomach muscles, painful lower-back problems and bad posture. It can also help you to build a firmer, better-looking body, as many famous filmstars and actresses are finding out.

The best way to improve your strength and tone your muscles is by working with weights. That way you add stress to an exercise so the body has to work harder, and you need to do fewer repeats to make it effective. Try it out at a gym or health club if you have the opportunity. There you will find special machines and have access to barbells and instructors. At home, you can always do exercises with home-made or bought weights. To make your own, fill 2 socks with sand, weighing them to get the right amount, then tie the socks tightly just above the level of the sand. Or make weights out of empty plastic bottles or containers. A little water added to the sand will increase the weight.

Start using the lightest weights and only progress to heavier ones when you are ready for them. Never exercised before? Start with no more than 0.25–0.5-kg (½–1-lb) weights. Stronger starter? You may be able to use 1–1.5-kg (2–3-lb) weights. One famous filmstar amazed the guests at a health spa with her leg and thigh work-outs, exercising each leg 50 times with 3-lb weights tied to her ankles! Not something to emulate unless you are truly fit and strong, or well supervised. Always start off gently. You are not in a race. Do not strain yourself. And as with any exercise, consult your doctor first if necessary and particularly if you have high blood pressure or heart problems.

Begin with warm ups, then do each exercise 5 or 6 times. After you have been doing them for several weeks, progress to 10 times. When you can do the exercises easily, you can try slightly heavier weights. Really fit people can handle 4.5–7-kg (10–15-lb) weights.

The pendulum
Very good for your ribcage, upper arms and stomach. Lie flat on the floor, legs together and straight. Hold one weight with both hands at the level of your upper thighs. Keeping your arms straight, lift the weight up and backwards until your arms are stretched out on the floor behind your head. Don't jerk – move smoothly and slowly.

Arm signals
Good for pectoral muscles. Stand upright, legs together, holding weights straight out in front of you. Open your arms wide, then return to first position.

Tummy tenser
Lie flat on the floor, with your feet anchored under a piece of furniture. Hold one weight between your hands near your chin. Try to raise your head and shoulders off the ground to a sitting position without using your hands for support.

The yo-yo
For strengthening arms. Stand up straight with your back against a wall, holding a weight in each hand at your sides. Bend your right elbow and lift a weight to your shoulder, turning your wrist outwards. Slowly lower the weight and repeat with the other arm.

Weight crouch
Good for hips, legs and abdomen. Stand, legs slightly apart, back straight, with weights held at your waist. Rise on to your toes, then slowly crouch down, opening your legs and bending your knees. Slowly return to a standing position.

Chin pull
Stand with your feet slightly apart, a weight held high in each hand at shoulder height, elbows bent. Crouch down and take weights down with you to the floor. Straighten up, bringing weights to chin level again.

Bench press
For shoulders and chest. Lie on a hard wooden bench or a hard bed, with your legs hanging over the edge, feet flat on the floor. Hold a weight in each hand, elbows bent, resting on your chest. Lift your arms, straightening your elbows; gently lower them.

The pendulum ▶

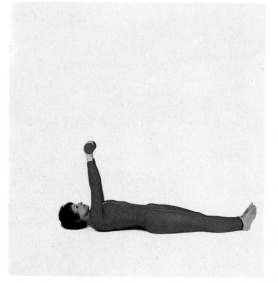
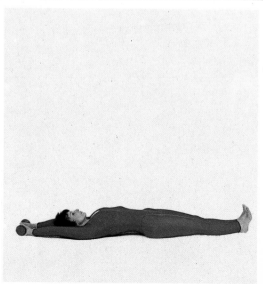

Arm signals ▶ **Tummy tenser** ▶

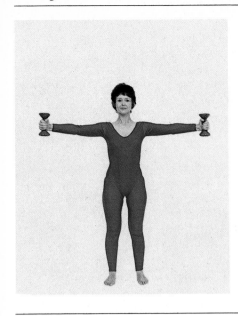 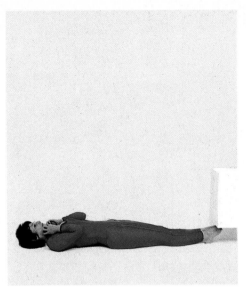 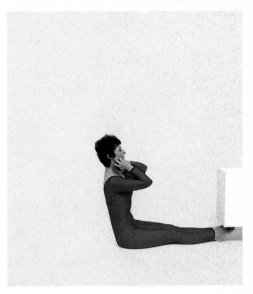

The yo-yo ▶ **Weight crouch** ▶

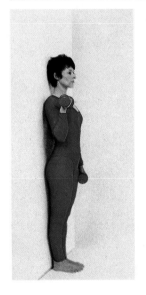 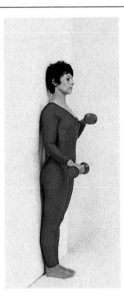 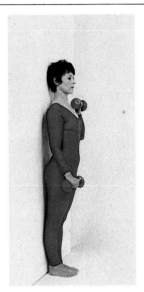 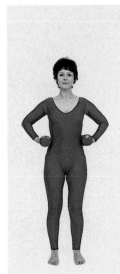 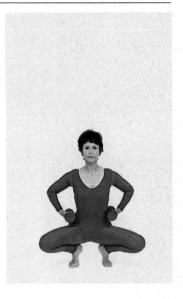

Chin pull ▶ **Bench press** ▶

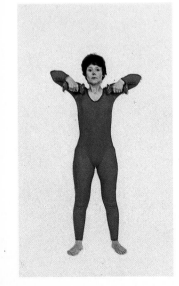 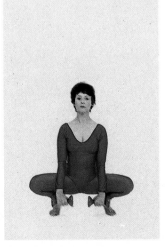 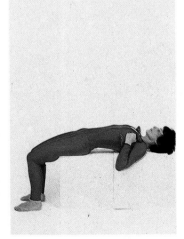 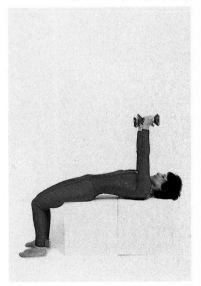

Yoga

The cult of yoga goes back thousands of years. The word yoga comes from the Sanskrit language and means harmony or union. That is what it gives you – a harmony of mind and body. Unlike other exercise regimes, yoga aims to calm the mind as well as improve suppleness, and it can be done by people of any age because it is done slowly. You do not have to be an athlete but you do need to practise regularly, gradually stretching your muscles and tuning your body.

Although originally an Eastern cult embracing philosophy, diet and meditation as well as exercise, Hatha Yoga, the physical discipline, is now practised by people all over the world. The asanas (body postures) are designed for each part of the body and consist of slow, controlled movements. Yogis, those who practise yoga, aim to have better control over their physical selves in order to leave their minds free to meditate. In our stressful modern society, yoga has a place in relieving tension and achieving tranquillity.

Do not hurry your exercises. Go into each particular posture slowly, concentrating hard, taking about 10–15 seconds from the start to your final position. Once you are there, hold for as long as comfort allows. The final phase of any exercise is a slow return to the original position . . . always the emphasis on slowness, concentration and control. After completing each asana, relax completely.

As a beginner you may be able to hold a pose no longer than 5 seconds, but you can increase your holding time by about 5 seconds a week as you become more efficient. As you gradually build up more strength and suppleness you can increase the scope of the exercises you do. Always do yoga in complete silence, and always be sure to go to the toilet before you begin. Your body must be completely relaxed.

Breathing Exercises

Breath control is an important part of yoga and very beneficial. Always breathe through your nose, and when practising breathing exercises do so out-of-doors or in front of an open window.

1 Sit in a comfortable position, with your back straight, and close your left nostril with your finger. Inhale slowly and deeply through the other nostril, counting to 4. Now close the right nostril with your thumb, retaining your breath for a count of between 1 and 4 seconds.

Open the left nostril and exhale, taking between 4–8 seconds to empty the lungs – the longer the better. Breathe in through the left nostril to a count of 4, close the nostril again and hold for a count of 1–4 seconds before slowly exhaling through the right nostril for 4–8 seconds. Repeat the exercise about 5 times.

When you inhale, concentrate on expanding your ribcage, pushing out your abdomen. When you exhale, pull in your abdomen as much as possible.

2 Sit up straight in a chair and inhale through your nose, breathing deeply. Take about 5 seconds to fill your lower lungs, expanding your ribs and pushing the abdomen out. Then fill the top of your lungs for about 5 seconds, expanding your chest and tightening your abdomen. Hold for 1–4 seconds and exhale slowly and completely.

3 Sit up straight. First empty your lungs completely to remove the stale air by breathing in through the nose and out through the mouth, pulling in the diaphragm. Relax your arms. Inhale very slowly through your nose, counting to 8, pushing out your chest and abdomen. At the same time, raise your arms. If you do this exercise standing, rise onto your toes. Hold, then relax, exhaling slowly. Repeat about 5 times.

The crocodile ▶

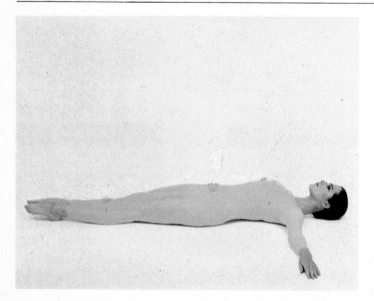

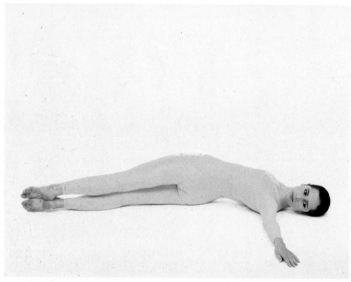

Yoga Movements

The dead pose

This has to be the easiest exercise of all! Start and finish off each yoga session by lying flat on the floor, legs straight, arms at sides, trying to relax every muscle in your body. Have your palms upturned and breathe rhythmically. Close your eyes and try to relax your mind as well as your body. Try muscle-tightening and letting-go when you have the time. This consists of tensing and then relaxing the muscles in each part of the body in turn, starting with your right toes.

Think of your eyes being deep inside your head and feel as though you can see out of the back of your skull. If someone lifts your hand, it should be so relaxed it is floppy. Stay like this for 2 minutes.

The cobra

An exercise for the pectoral muscles which support the breasts; also good for the chin, neck and back. Relieves tension. Lie face down, elbows bent so that your hands are resting palms down on the floor, near your shoulders and chin. Rest your forehead on the floor. Slowly raise your head, straightening your arms, so your spine is curved but your navel touches the ground. You do not have to straighten out your arms completely if it is not comfortable. Tilt your head back and hold for about 10 seconds. Gradually work up to 30 as you get better at it. Gently lower yourself down. Repeat twice.

The crocodile

This exercise aids suppleness of the spine. Do it smoothly. Lie on your back on the floor, arms extended at shoulder height, feet together. Inhale, keeping your shoulders flat to the floor, turning your head to the left and twisting your spine, hips, legs and feet to the right. In a continuous movement, and holding your breath, twist the other way. Return to starting position and exhale. Repeat 3 times.

The stick position

Stretches sides and waist and tones arms, legs and back. Lie on your back on the floor with your arms stretched over your head. Inhale and stretch out your whole body, feeling yourself fully extended. Exhale and release the stretch. Contract the muscles on either side of your spine, pressing the small of your back into the floor. Hold for count of 5 and relax. Repeat 3–4 times.

The cobra ▶

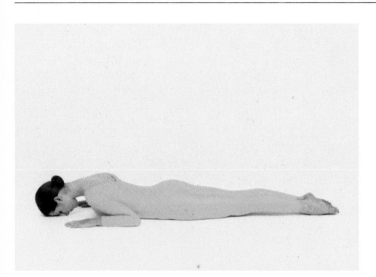

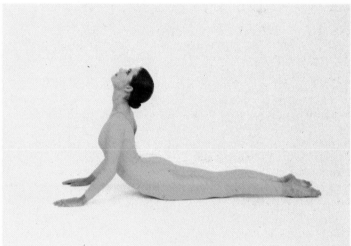

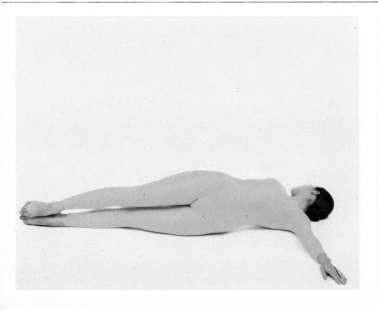

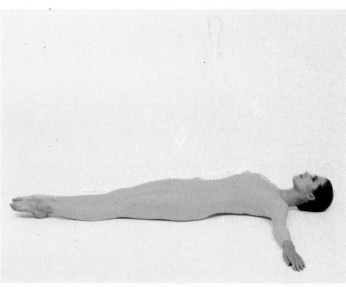

Pose of a child

This is wonderful if you feel edgy, cramped or tired. Kneel on the floor, sitting back on your heels, your hands pointing back. Slowly bend forward and lower your head until your forehead touches the floor in front of your knees. As you do this, bring your arms gently back, palms up, so they rest on the floor beside your body. Relax with your chest against your knees. Hold for as long as you feel comfortable.

The cat

Good for your back and abdominal muscles. Kneel on all fours on the floor, your hands and knees parallel, and bend your head down. Your spine should arch like an angry cat. Do deep breathing, pulling the abdomen in and up with each exhalation. Inhale, hollowing the back, raising your head.

A variation is to kneel on all fours and lower your chest to the floor, with your weight on your arms. Hold for about 5 seconds. Return to first all-fours position and arch your back like an angry cat. Hold for 5 seconds. Relax. Now lift one leg and bring it towards your head. Touch it, if possible, and hold for 5 seconds. Then lift your head up and back and stretch the lifted leg outwards, raising it high but keeping it straight. Arms should be straight, too. Hold. Now return your leg slowly to your head and hold. Relax. Repeat with other leg. Do complete exercise all over again.

Pose of a child ▶

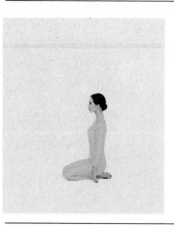 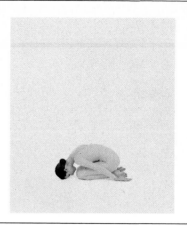

The cat ▶

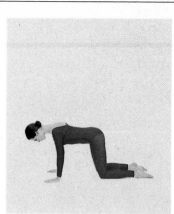

The cat variation ▶

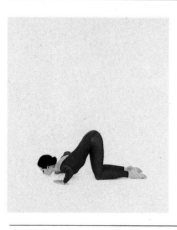 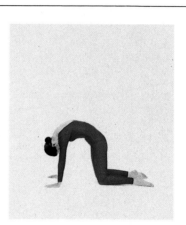 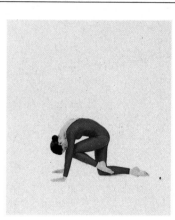

Knee rocks ▶

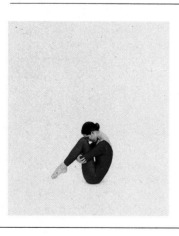 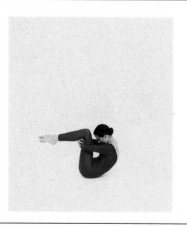 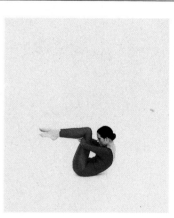

The camel ▶

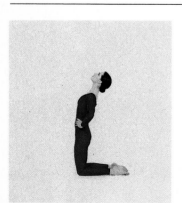 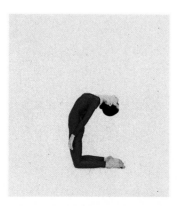 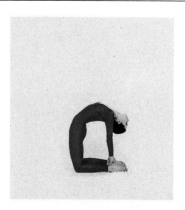

The plough ▶

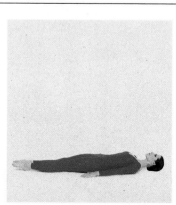

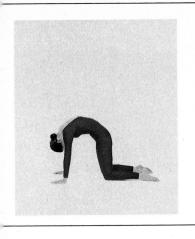
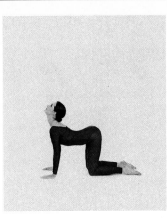

Knee rocks

Sit on the floor with your knees bent, clasping your hands *under* your knees. Bring your head as close to your knees as possible. Rock gently back onto your spine, with back rounded, legs together. Rock back and forth rhythmically about 12 times. If you like, start the exercise from your back rather than the sitting position.

Knee and thigh stretch

Tones inner thigh muscles, helps to stop leg stiffness and flabbiness. Sit straight on the floor and bend your knees, bringing the soles of your feet together and close to your body. Clasp your hands firmly round your feet and pull them towards you, flattening your knees and thighs to the ground as much as possible without straining. Hold for at least 5 seconds. Relax and repeat 3 times. Don't worry if your knees will not reach the floor – with practise they eventually will.

The camel

(Gentle, OK for anyone past middle age.) This makes your spine more flexible and improves posture and rounded shoulders. Kneel on the floor, legs together, back straight, toes pointing backwards. Put your hands on your waist and bend slowly backwards, your pelvis pushing forward. Lift your chin and let your head hang back and your hands hang down. When you are more supple, you can try to touch your feet. Clench your buttocks and push your thighs

and pelvis forward as you lean. Hold for 5 seconds, and increase holding time as you become more supple.

The plough

Marvellous for the spine, good for stomach muscles, thighs and hips. Lie on your back on the floor with your arms at your sides, palms down, legs stretched out straight and together. Lift your legs slowly, pushing down on your hands, and bring your legs over your head. When they are vertical, give the small of your back some support with your hands. Now try to touch the floor behind you with your toes, keeping your knees straight and moving your legs very slowly. This is very difficult unless you are extremely supple. Hold the pose for as long as comfortable, then very carefully move your legs back to the original position, and relax.

Spread and stretch

Sit on the floor with your legs spread wide apart. (If you are very supple, the best way to reach this position is to do a split.) Place your hands on your legs near your knees and, bending forward from the waist, bring your head down towards the floor. Stretch as far as you can, hold for 10 seconds, relax and repeat twice more.

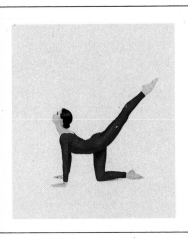
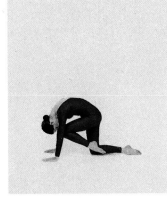

Knee and thigh stretch ▶

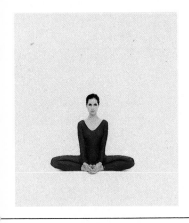
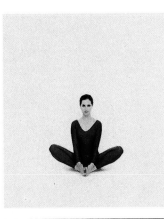

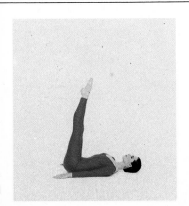
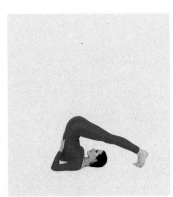

Spread and stretch ▶

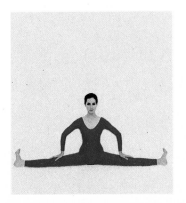
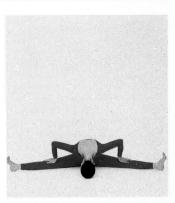

Dancing

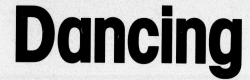

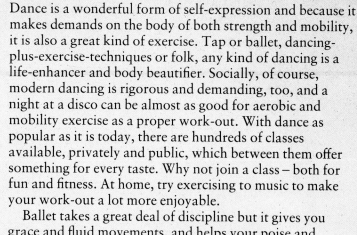

Dance is a wonderful form of self-expression and because it makes demands on the body of both strength and mobility, it is also a great kind of exercise. Tap or ballet, dancing-plus-exercise-techniques or folk, any kind of dancing is a life-enhancer and body beautifier. Socially, of course, modern dancing is rigorous and demanding, too, and a night at a disco can be almost as good for aerobic and mobility exercise as a proper work-out. With dance as popular as it is today, there are hundreds of classes available, privately and public, which between them offer something for every taste. Why not join a class – both for fun and fitness. At home, try exercising to music to make your work-out a lot more enjoyable.

Ballet takes a great deal of discipline but it gives you grace and fluid movements, and helps your poise and posture. Your kicks, bends and leaps will have grand-sounding names like grands battements, pliés, jetés, sissonnées, ports de bras and arabesques. Barre-work helps you with leg exercises. After two weeks, you'll feel some improvement, but it will take about six months to see a change of shape. It's well worth the effort. Beginners classes can leave you stiff if you haven't done exercise too often, but the aching subsides the more exercises you do.

Disco dancing isn't as good as modern dancing and ballet for limbering up but it is an aerobic exercise which builds stamina and burns up calories.

Modern dance routines exercise every part of your body. Try this at home: Sit on the floor with one leg bent in front and one behind. Sit up straight and raise your arms. Stretch from the waist and do graceful sweeps to the side, around and down, brushing the floor in front, making one continuous sweeping circular motion.

Jazz ballet is much more free, releases your inhibitions and gives your pelvis and hips a good work-out.

Tap dancing fulfills your fantasies, gives you a marvellous sense of accomplishment and is a fun way to shape up.

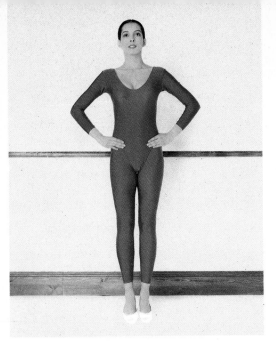
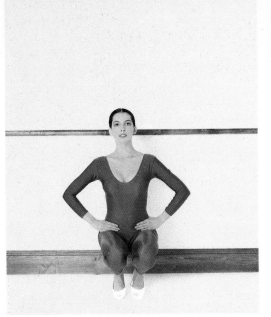

Exercises

1 Do knee bends for ankles, thighs and lower back. Stand with your feet together and hands lightly on your hips. Rise on your toes and do a deep knee bend *very* slowly. Straighten up, bend again slowly, then lower your heels. Repeat 20 times. Do each section of the exercise to a beat of four.

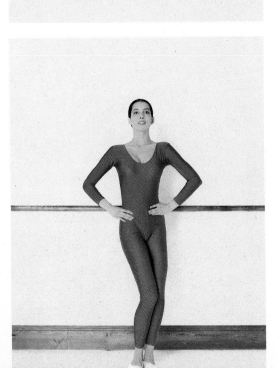
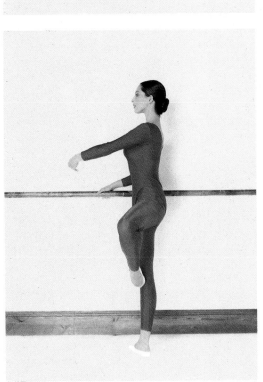
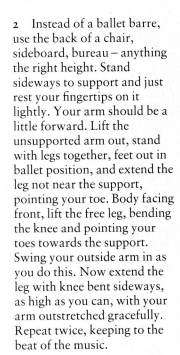

2 Instead of a ballet barre, use the back of a chair, sideboard, bureau – anything the right height. Stand sideways to support and just rest your fingertips on it lightly. Your arm should be a little forward. Lift the unsupported arm out, stand with legs together, feet out in ballet position, and extend the leg not near the support, pointing your toe. Body facing front, lift the free leg, bending the knee and pointing your toes towards the support. Swing your outside arm in as you do this. Now extend the leg with knee bent sideways, as high as you can, with your arm outstretched gracefully. Repeat twice, keeping to the beat of the music.

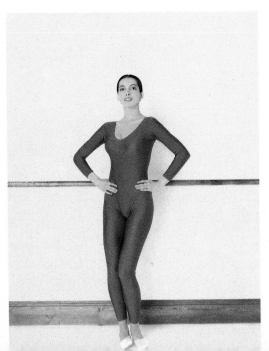
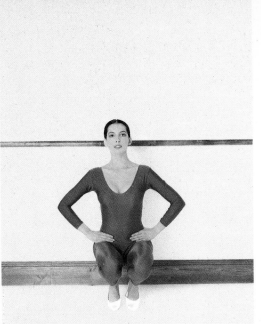

3 For a trim waist, stand with your feet together and arms loosely by your sides or lightly on your hips. Keeping your knees together, bend them slightly. Swing them to the left and then to the right, keeping to a firm brisk beat. Keep the top half of your body facing the front so that you twist at the waist. Repeat 20 times.

67

Running

Jogging – sometimes referred to as the art of running with your brakes on – has become more than just a passing craze. Running is really a simple form of exercise and can be done, more or less, by most of us, whatever our age. You don't have to join a club to do it, nor do you need to spend a great deal on equipment and gear.

Running is extremely effective in improving the efficiency of your heart, increasing lung power, toning muscles (particularly leg) and improving blood circulation. It helps to reduce stress and plays a great part in improving your all-round physical fitness. Devotees say it even increases your self-esteem.

You can jog alone or in company, at any time of the day, and for whatever distance you wish. Of course, you should not over-do your exertion. You're not aiming to win Olympic medals or prove anything to anybody.

Your running *speed* has little effect on the number of calories you burn – weight counts more than pace. For instance, a 220-lb person would use 150 calories running a mile, while a 120-lb person would only burn 82. If you ran 5 miles a day (at a weight of 180 lbs) you would lose about a pound in weight every 5–6 days, without changing your eating pattern! Running combined with a diet is an extremely effective way of losing weight.

If you have never done more than run for the bus before, here's how to begin. First of all, don't worry about speed. Just move along easily and stop when you get tired. Never strain yourself. Build up your stamina first. A 20-minute jog three times a week is enough to keep you healthy and fit.

Week 1: Try some brisk walking.

Week 2: Begin by walking for 10 minutes. Break into a jog for about 50 yards, then slow down to walking pace again.

Week 3: Continue walks but with two or three 50- or 100-yard jogs breaking them up.

Week 4: Take a walk and jog for 100 yards. Do alternative walking/jogging. If you feel out of breath for longer than two minutes after stopping, take it slower.

Week 5: Continue to build up to jogging for the whole 20 minutes.

Repeated running brings improvement in your condition and stamina. You have to keep it up. But you don't need to take on more than you wish. Little and more often is better than straining once in a while.

What can go wrong? Over-doing running could result in ligament strain, knee and back injuries and inflamed tendons, in addition to blisters and other aches and pains. You can get Jogger's Kidney, where blood leaks into the urine (brought on by exertion; it clears up with rest but do see your doctor) or Jogger's Nipple, caused by the friction of blouse and bouncing, unprotected breasts. Keen runners prevent it with strips of plaster or special bras.

Joggers' Guide

● Get your doctor's permission to run if you are more than two stone overweight, over 35, have a family history of heart disease, suffer

from high blood pressure or are recovering from illness.

● Warm up your muscles first. See exercises.

● Do not go jogging up to three hours after eating a heavy meal or taking a hot bath. Wait half an hour after waking up.

● Stop immediately if you feel dizzy or nauseous, develop cramp, chest pains, or uncomfortable breathlessness.

● Good supportive, well-fitting running shoes which have enough room for your toes to lie straight are a good idea if you intend to run regularly. If you run a mile, each of your shoes lands on the ground about 1000 times. A good running shoe should be flexible, especially at the ball of the foot, and should have a fairly hard sole with a layer of soft cushioning between it and the foot. You don't need spikes.

● Socks are probably more hygienic than bare feet. Choose cotton or wool, which will soak up sweat. Don't buy them so tight that they restrict toes or so loose that they may cause blisters.

● You can run in any clothes you wish, but most people find easy clothes such as track suits or shorts best.

● Keep your toenails trimmed. If your nails are too long, they take a beating in shoes.

Running is an ideal exercise. It's invigorating, free, and can be done as easily in a busy city as in the country

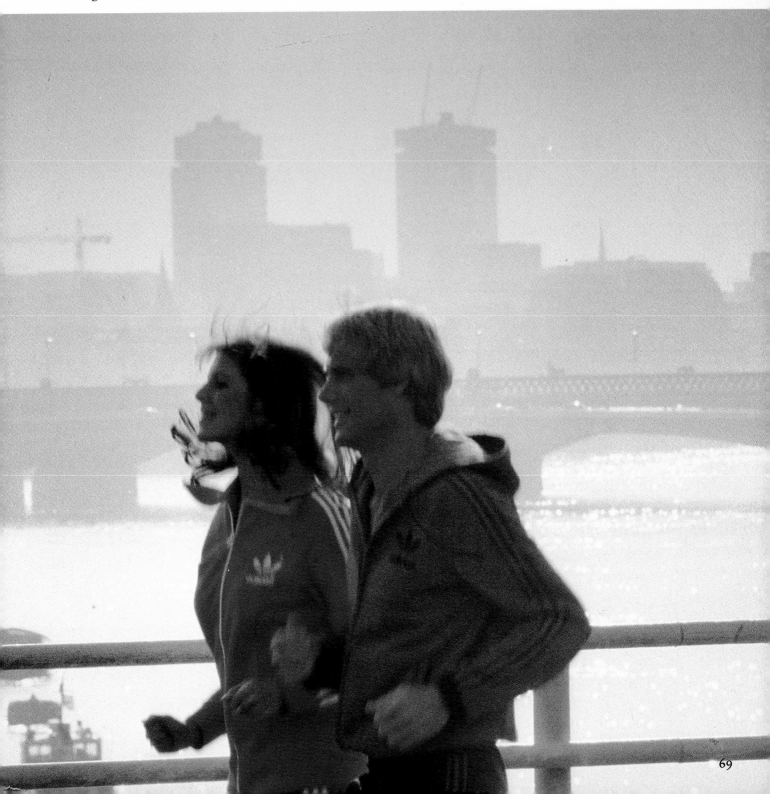

Sporting Ways

Sport is fun and enjoyable, and above all, it's a great aid to fitness. It tones you up, gives you a healthy glow, relaxes you and can become an absorbing and rewarding part of your life. The table opposite outlines the benefits of some popular sports. Bear in mind the message of all the exercise sections: build up slowly, exercise consistently, stop if you feel faint, exhausted or simply too strained. Sports, like all good exercise, are to be enjoyed!

SPORT	HEALTH BENEFITS	BEAUTY BENEFITS	CALORIES USED	COMMENT
Cycling	If you work hard at it cycling is good exercise for your cardio-respiratory system. It is also relaxing, and helps flexibility.	Improves thigh muscles and firms buttocks.	At 24 km (15 miles) per hour you could use up about 650 calories in an hour. At 16 km (10 miles) per hour this drops to 390; at 8 km (5 miles) to 240.	It's fun, faster than walking and builds up stamina of heart and lungs provided you push hard enough, for long enough.
Golf	A great relaxer, golf helps you to unwind and get rid of tension. It's a non-strenuous, gentle exercise with a lot of walking.	Quite good for flexibility of arms and legs. Allows you to get lots of fresh air.	About 200–240 calories an hour.	Not a sport to improve endurance or muscular development. Benefits are probably more psychological than physical.
Riding	Good for overall fitness and legs, thighs and buttocks. Relaxing and good tension-easer.	Improves grace and deportment.	A gentle trot will obviously use less energy than a canter – but the horse does most of the work so you won't expend many calories.	Moderate/low energy expenditure on the whole, but can be invigorating and satisfying.
Roller skating	A good exercise for heart and lungs.	Helps tone and trim thighs, calves, buttocks, waist and hips.	About 360 an hour.	Great fun – especially roller-disco. Make sure your boots and skates fit.
Sailing	Dinghy sailing is a hard physical sport. It quickens reactions, and exercises back, legs and stomach. Cruising is much softer; it doesn't call for so much exertion.	Makes you look healthier, but if you don't want to look weather-beaten, use a strong protective sunscreen.	Up to 400 calories in a more strenuous hour.	Not recommended if you have a weak back. You need to train properly and you must be able to swim 45 metres (50 yards) in light clothing, to sail with a reputable club.
Squash	Excellent for stamina and very good for suppleness. Helps work off frustrations. Provides good muscle work-out.	Relaxing – because it works off tensions, you feel and look more at ease. Helps suppleness.	In half an hour, the usual length of play, you could use up as many as 300 calories.	Fast and furious, squash can be exciting. It may be expensive, and you need to book courts well in advance.
Swimming	An all-over body toner, swimming develops stamina, suppleness and strength. Good exercise for older people, or those with rheumatism or arthritis, because the body is supported.	An excellent exercise for the pectoral muscles supporting the breasts. Breaststroke is good for hips and knees; backstroke and crawl for shoulders and trunk.	280–700 per hour depending on intensity of effort.	Try a variety of different strokes to exercise different groups of muscles. Build up slowly to two or three 20-minute sessions weekly. Don't swim within two hours of a big meal.
Tennis	Develops balance, enhances alertness, strengthens hand/eye co-ordination. Unless played competitively to high standards, tennis does not really stretch the body significantly. Good exercise if you are out of condition.	Gives you an outdoor glow. The bending and stretching is good for your waist and legs, and makes arms and shoulders more supple.	200–400 an hour depending on how much you put into your game.	Good social sport for all ages, but not recommended if you have back trouble. To play it really well, you need to be an athlete. Even if you're not, however, it's great fun.
Water skiing	If you don't have strong thigh muscles, you'll need to develop them. An exhilarating sport in warm weather in a warm sea.	Toning for the legs, especially fronts of thighs, and back, shoulders and stomach muscles.	Probably not more than 60 calories in 10 minutes.	Not recommended if you have high blood pressure, heart problems, or if you are not at all fit.

Healthy Living

We all seem to be looking for magical solutions, whether it is a magic diet or a pill that solves our problems. But life, alas, is not as simple as all that. Today, looking good is looking healthy, looking vibrant and alive as if you were full of energy. This kind of energy does not come from taking extra vitamin pills. Good physical and emotional health, regular rest and exercise, a balanced diet, satisfying work and homelife . . . all these contribute.

Fatigue is caused by trying to cram too many things into a day. Combined with stress, and smoking, it leads to physical and mental overload. Recent research suggests that stress is a contributory factor to the present increase in the incidence of heart and blood vessel disease in both men and women.

It's true, of course, that we all have our survival levels and that stress can be stimulating as well as overwhelming. It is how you handle it that counts. Sedatives, uppers and downers, alcohol and drugs – even worry beads – are well-known remedies. Yet the best relaxers do not rely on drugs and medicines because you can get physical release from sports and exercise and calm and contentment from meditation and prayer.

Until the body screams for attention, we usually ignore it. When we do give it attention, it is often just for appearance's sake and not for health. Preventive Medicine, and now Prospective Medicine, help you to look at your own risk factors and work out a health-hazard appraisal.

For instance, if your family has had a run on cancer, diabetes or early coronaries, it would pay you to take more care of yourself and look more closely at the potential risk factors. If you smoke, make sure you have regular check-ups and chest examinations, especially after 20 years on cigarettes.

All women should regularly examine their breasts (leaflets on how to do this are freely available at local health clinics) and have regular check-ups, especially if there is any history of cancer in the family. If you have close relatives who died early from heart disease you should take extra care with your own diet and health, cutting down on hard fats, avoiding weighing more than recommended, and taking more physical exercise.

Foods we take for granted are suddenly coming into the spotlight of expert appraisal because of the possible health risk discovered by research. Expert committees on blood pressure, for instance, maintain that cutting our average daily intake of salt by half or more could have a significant effect on the overall incidence of high blood pressure. In the West, we use about half an ounce a day – not just at the table, because many convenience foods also contain it. Tea and coffee, known for their mildly stimulating effect because of the caffeine they contain, are also coming under scrutiny because some reports on people with coronary heart disease say that on average they have taken more cups of coffee than unaffected people. Too much caffeine causes sleeplessness and 'hypes' you up so much that you feel strained.

For better health you should eat less sugar, too, more fibre, less fat, and fewer calories. Prevention is the best medicine of all and moderation in everything is the best advice if you want to live longer and look your best.

To stay more relaxed, you have to make an effort. Simple tension-relieving exercises are a good pick-me-up after a hard day:

Slowly roll your head around in a complete circle, first one way, then the other; or shrug your shoulders round for a little while. Get more sleep. Have a hot scented bath, listen to music, give yourself time to unwind. If you suffer from insomnia, that old standby warm milk may help. Try meditating – breathe deeply and slowly and concentrate all your attention, trying to shut your mind to stray thoughts, worries, niggles, extraneous noise.

Are You at Risk?

Heart disease is one of the major causes of death in the Western World and doctors say a lot of it can be prevented. These are the primary risk factors listed by the American Heart Association.

Family history If you have a blood relative who has had a heart attack before the age of 50, the odds are greater that you are at risk. Coronary heart disease apparently runs in families.

Stress Tension, stress and aggressive behaviour place a strain on the heart. If you are the type of person who never lets go, who plans and worries and pushes yourself continuously, your body's hormonal system will act as it has been programmed to do ever since the Stone Age – it will prepare your body for 'flight or

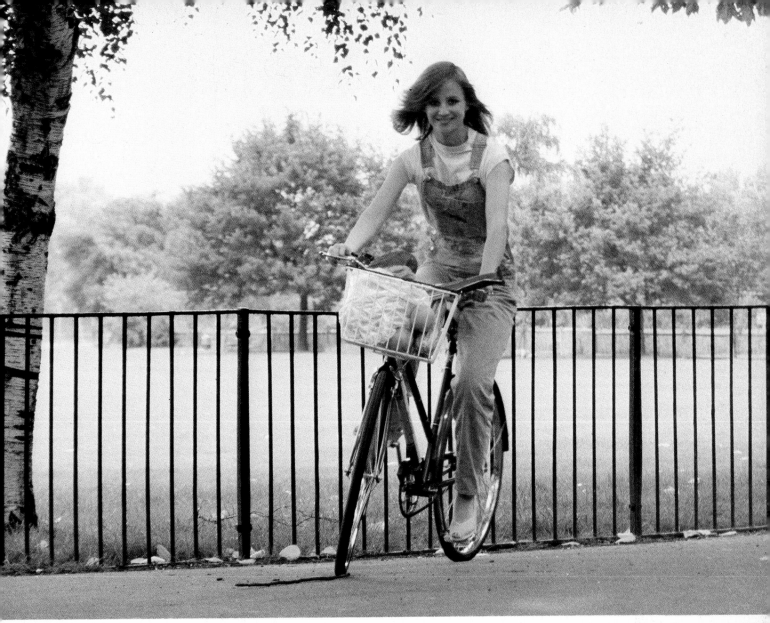

fight', speeding up your heart rate and increasing blood pressure. If you were either to physically run away or fight, your adrenal hormones would be burned up, and your tension would be consumed. But if you do neither and continue to look at life as looming threats and un-met challenges, your heart and pulmonary system will be under consistent pressure, which means excess wear-and-tear.

Inactivity　Sedentary people have more heart problems than those who are active.

High blood pressure　This is recognized as one of the major risk factors.

Obesity　Fat puts a strain on the heart because it has to squeeze blood through veins surrounded by fat deposits, and it has to cope with the extra strain of dragging more weight around.

Cigarettes　Smoking is now considered a major cause of heart disease. Carbon monoxide in the smoke – like that in car exhausts – diminishes the red blood cells' capacity to carry oxygen. Your heart will have to pump out more blood to get the same amount of oxygen through your body. The nicotine in cigarettes increases the flow of adrenalin, speeding up the heart rate and constricting blood vessels.

Cholesterol　If you have a high blood level of cholesterol, you should take action to reduce it. See pages 20 and 31.

Triglycerides　These are blood fats which are related to obesity. It will help if you lose weight. Cut down on dietary fats.

Diabetes　This is associated with an increased risk of heart disease.

Abnormal resting heart rate　A danger sign that can only be detected by your doctor.

The American Heart Association also lists three secondary risk factors: *Body build*: endomorphs (rounded) and mesomorphs (muscular) appear to be more at risk than ectomorphs (thin). *Your lung capacity*: The amount of air your lungs can hold appears to affect your heart. The more efficiently the lungs can oxygenate the blood, the less the demands on the heart. *Uric acid*: High levels lead to gout and those who suffer from it also are at risk from heart disease, especially if overweight.

Fresh air and regular exercise are as important to your well-being as the right kind of diet and the avoidance of drugs.

Beating the Baddies

You cannot be fit if you smoke, drink to excess, or take drugs. Nor are you fit if you are full of tension and strain. Life is hectic and full and we all need a crutch at some time or another, but when the crutch becomes a coffin, you are denying yourself both health and happiness.

Smoking

You must know the risks by now. But have they really registered? If you developed lung cancer and were forbidden to smoke, you would have to give it up, there and then. So why not do it now, before it becomes a reality.

The ritual of striking up is without doubt a suicide ritual, yet it is carried out by people all over the world, every hour of every day. This is what happens when you light up a cigarette.

● Smoke travels up the length of the cigarette and after about three lungfuls, particles of nicotine and tar begin to irritate the delicate tubules inside the lungs.

● The third toxic component in cigarette smoke, carbon monoxide, displaces oxygen in the blood and aggravates heart disease.

● Particles of nicotine and tar start to coat the bronchial tubes with an oily thick tar, forcing the lungs to produce phlegm. Your smokers' cough is an attempt by the lungs to get rid of the irritation.

● The last puffs on your cigarette are saturated with chemicals and irritants, coating the lungs with more liquid tar, causing more irritation and phlegm.

● When the mixture of tar and phlegm becomes infected it congeals and festers in your lungs, obstructing the air flow.

● Nicotine constricts blood vessels, raises blood pressure.

● Smoking reduces the blood supply to the womb in pregnant women, causing the placenta to contract. Babies of women who smoke are on average 200g (7 oz) lighter than those of non-smokers. Carbon monoxide from the mother's circulation is taken up and to some extent concentrated in the baby's blood, reducing the amount of oxygen available to the baby.

The risks

Smoking can lead to cancer of the larynx and lung cancer. In Britain about 100 people a day die from lung cancer, six times the number who die on the roads, and half the victims are under 65. Smokers are 70 times more likely to develop lung cancer than non-smokers and are also liable to get cancer of the bladder and the mouth. Tar is the cause of lung cancer and of lung damage leading to chronic bronchitis and emphysema.

Bronchitis starts as a smokers' cough. As the air tubes and sacs get damaged by smoke, the lungs cannot get enough air and the blood cannot therefore get the oxygen the body needs to function normally. Crippled by breathlessness, unable to walk far or climb stairs, and in the end unable to work at all, the victim becomes disabled, prematurely retired; and there is a strong risk of premature death.

If cancer and bronchitis don't get a smoker, heart problems can. The risk increases with smoking – you are twice as likely to have heart problems as non-smokers; up to five times as likely in the 35–44 group. Carbon monoxide is particularly hazardous to someone who already suffers from a bad heart. The effect of one cigarette increases the heartbeat from about 77 beats a minute to 88 beats a minute, blood pressure increases, fats in the blood increase in concentration and all these factors lead to the accumulation of fatty deposits in the arteries.

Giving up

You can do a Cold Turkey and just not buy any more cigarettes. Or you can try to wean yourself off smoking gradually, turning to the low-tar, low-nicotine, low-carbon monoxide brands, and cutting down the number of cigarettes you smoke each day. There must be as many smoking cures as there are brands, but in the end, it is just your willpower that matters. You must try to care passionately. Disgusting, dirty, unpleasant . . . those are the words you must think of every time you go to a cigarette machine.

What about substitutes? Does giving up smoking make you eat more? Not necessarily. Smoking does destroy a lot of your taste and when you actually begin to savour food again, you increase your appetite. But you do not need to gain weight and you can always take up some low-calorie alternative, such as chewing gum, if you need oral satisfaction.

Half measures are better than none. But make sure yours lead to giving up altogether.

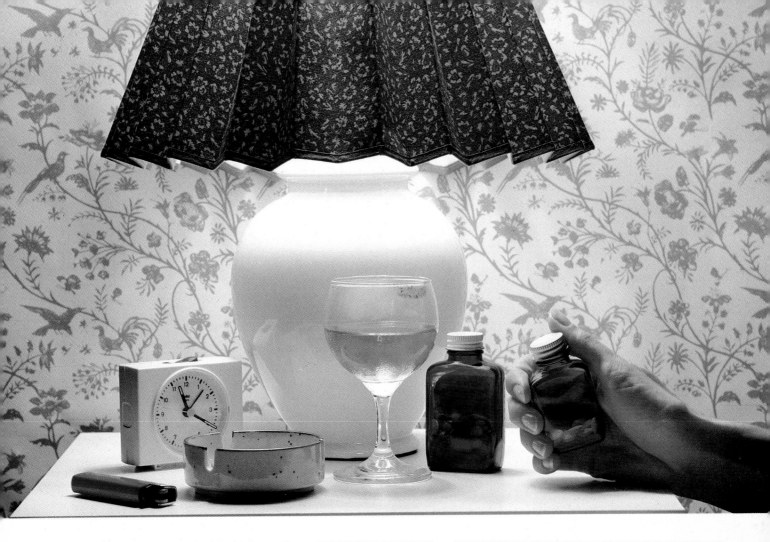

Cigarettes, alcohol and pills of all sorts are a trio tolerated by most but inherently dangerous to many. Cut down on your intake, or cut them out all together.

Alcohol

Drinking is a social habit and therefore a pleasurable activity, but when it becomes a problem – an addiction – it can ruin your health and your life. Dependence on alcohol interferes with work, homelife and pleasures and, if unchecked, can lead to chronic ill health and death. When does a social drinker become an alcoholic? The barrier can be very fine and it is hard to admit you have broken it. You have problems if you neglect food for drink; you have to drink *every* day; you turn to drink for consolation from stress and worries; you drive under the influence of drink; you have bouts of bad memory because of drinking; you have a 'morning after' every morning; you hide drink around the house; you are unable to stop drinking; you do not know when you have had enough but go on and make a nuisance of yourself; you drink alone. If any of these apply to you, you are technically in danger.

There's a long distance between social drinking, becoming dependent on drink and becoming an alcoholic. But it is as well to recognize the symptoms so you can stop the rot before it gets any worse.

Drugs

Do you rely on a pill to get you through? Do you take pills of some kind every day, even though they are not prescribed by your doctor? We are pill-prone, with easy access to pills to cure almost every malaise of modern life, whether it is stress or lack of sleep, too much adrenalin or too little. If you find yourself taking some kind of pill every day and you do not have an illness that necessitates taking any, it might be a good idea to take a step back and ask yourself why? Perhaps it is not a pill you need but a change of life-style. For instance, if you feel you need to take pills for constipation, perhaps you should try to introduce more fibre into your diet, eat more wholemeal cereals and bran instead. If you take pills to get to sleep, perhaps a course of exercise, running or yoga would do the trick more healthily. If stress in life makes you feel you cannot do without tranquillizers, you need to re-think the way you live. Perhaps you need to change your job or your surroundings.

Pills have their place. But you should not rely on them for a constant crutch. Attack the cause of the problem, not the result.

Calorie counter and nutrition tables

In the following tables all vegetables are boiled unless otherwise stated. Carbohydrates per 25g (1oz) or per portion are occasionally omitted where inappropriate, e.g. tea, parsley.

CU = Carbohydrate Units per 25g (1oz) unless other quantity stated. 5 grams of carbohydrate is equivalent to 1 CU.

Tr. = Trace   ea. = each   sl. = slice   pce. = piece   car. = carton

FOOD OR DRINK	CALORIES per 25g (1oz)	CALORIES PER AVERAGE PORTION	PROTEIN PERCENTAGE	FAT PERCENTAGE	Cu PER 25g (1oz) unless portion stated	CARBOHYDRATE PERCENTAGE
Almonds, shelled	161	about 10 each 15ml (1tbs): 30	16.9	53.5	0	4.3
flaked and ground						
Apples	10	medium-sized: 40	0.2	Tr.	2 ea.	9.2
juice	13	115ml (4fl oz): 52	0.1	0	¾	12.0
stewed with a little sugar	19	115g (4oz): 76	0.3	Tr.	1	17.3
Apricots, fresh	7	115g (4oz): 28	0.5	Tr.	¼	6.2
canned	30	½ small can: 110	0.5	Tr.	1½	27.7
dried	52	about 26 each	4.8	Tr.	2½	43.4
stewed without sugar	19	115g (4oz): 76	1.8	Tr.	1	16.1
Artichoke, globe	4	medium-sized: 20	1.1	Tr.	0	2.7
Jerusalem	5	115g (4oz): 20	1.6	Tr.	0	3.2
Asparagus	5	140g (5oz): 25	3.4	Tr.	0	1.1
Aubergine, fried	60	140g (5oz): 300	0.7	Tr.+	0	3.1
Avocado	64	½ medium-sized: 320	4.2	22.2	½:½	1.8
Bacon						
gammon, boiled	77	85g (3oz): 230	24.7	18.9	0	0
rashers, fried						
back	133	2 rashers: 195	24.9	40.6	0	0
streaky	142	3 rashers: 225	23.1	44.8	0	0
rashers, grilled						
back	116	2 rashers: 128	25.3	33.8	0	0
gammon	65	2 rashers: 200	29.5	12.2	0	0
streaky	120	3 rashers: 126	24.5	36.0	0	0
Bananas	22	medium-sized: 80	1.1	0.3	4 ea.	19.2
Barley, boiled	34		2.7	0.6	1½	27.6
Bass, steamed	36	140g (5oz): 180	19.5	5.1	0	0
Beans						
baked	18	140g (5oz) can: 90	5.1	0.5	½	10.3
broad	14	115g (4oz): 56	4.1	0.6	½	7.1
butter	27	25g (1oz): 27	7.1	0.3	1	17.1
French	2	115g (4oz): 8	0.8	Tr.	0	1.1
haricot	26	115g (4oz): 104	6.6	0.5	1	16.6
runner	5	115g (4oz): 20	1.9	0.2	0	2.7
Beansprouts	2	115g (4oz): 8	1.6	Tr.	0	0.8
Beef						
brisket, boiled	93	115g (4oz): 372	27.6	23.9	0	0
corned	62	3 slices: 170	26.9	12.1	0	0
minced, stewed	65	115g (4oz): 260	23.1	15.2	0	0
rib, roast	100	115g (4oz): 400	22.4	28.8	0	0
rump steak, grilled	62	170g (6oz): 372	27.3	12.1	0	0
sirloin roast	81	115g (4oz): 324	23.6	21.1	0	0
stewing steak	64	115g (4oz): 256	30.9	11.0	0	0
topside, roast (lean)	61	115g (4oz): 244	26.6	12.0	0	0

FOOD OR DRINK	CALORIES per 25g (1oz)	CALORIES PER AVERAGE PORTION	PROTEIN PERCENTAGE	FAT PERCENTAGE	Cu PER 25g (1oz) unless portion stated	CARBOHYDRATE PERCENTAGE
Beef extract	50	15ml (1 tbs): 10	39.1	0.7	0	2.9
Beer					(pint)	
ale, brown, bottled	8	560ml (pint): 160	0.3	Tr.	8	3.0
ale, pale, bottled	9	560ml (pint): 180	0.3	Tr.	8	2.0
ale, strong	20	560ml (pint): 400	0.7	Tr.	18½	6.1
bitter, canned	9	560ml (pint): 180	0.3	Tr.	9	2.3
bitter, draught	9	560ml (pint): 180	0.3	Tr.	9	2.3
lager, bottled	8	560ml (pint): 160	0.2	Tr.	8	1.5
mild, draught	7	560ml (pint): 140	0.2	Tr.	7	1.6
stout, bottled	10	560ml (pint): 200	0.3	Tr.	10	4.2
Beetroot	12	3 slices: 30	1.8	Tr.	½	9.9
Biscuits						
cream crackers	126	40 each	9.5	16.3	1 ea.	68.3
crispbread, rye	92	30–35 each	9.4	2.1	1 ea.	70.6
starch reduced, wheat		20–25 each	45.3	7.6	½ ea.	36.9
digestive, chocolate	141	80–130 each	6.8	24.1	2 ea.	66.5
digestive, plain	134	60–70 each	9.8	20.5	1½ ea.	66.0
ginger nuts	130	35 each	5.6	15.2	1½ ea.	79.1
oatcakes	126	55–90 each	10.0	18.3	2 ea.	63.0
sandwich	146	65–80 each	5.0	25.9	2 ea.	69.2
shortbread	144	40–70 each	6.2	26.0	3½ ea.	65.5
water biscuits	126	30 each	10.8	12.5	1 ea.	75.8
Blackberries	8	85g (3oz): 24	1.3	Tr.	½	6.4
stewed with little sugar	17	115g (4oz): 68	1.1	Tr.	1	14.8
Blackcurrants	8	85g (3oz): 24	0.9	Tr.	½	6.6
cordial (undiluted)	65	average glass: 30	0.1	0	3½	60.9
stewed with little sugar	17	115g (4oz): 68	0.8	Tr.	1	15.0
Bloater, grilled	53	2 medium-sized: 245	17.4	12.9	0	0
Brains, boiled						
calf's	43	115g (4oz): 172	12.7	11.2	0	0
lamb's	36	115g (4oz): 144	11.6	8.8	0	0
Bran	59	15ml (1tbs): 10	14.1	5.5	1½	26.8
cereal	78	small bowl: 90	15.1	5.7	2½	43.0
Brawn	44	55g (2oz): 88	12.4	11.5	0	0
Brazil nuts	177	about 20 each	10.9	64.0	0	5.2
Bread						
brown	64	small slice: 66	8.9	2.7	2	44.7
currant	71	small slice: 71	6.4	4.4	3	51.8
malt	71	small slice: 75	8.3	3.3	3	49.4
rolls:						
brown, crusty	82	small roll: 144	11.5	3.2	5 ea.	57.2
white, crusty	83	small roll: 145	11.6	3.2	5 ea.	57.2
starch-reduced	110	25 each	44.0	4.1	½ ea.	45.7
slimmers' (per slice)		35–45	10.0	2.6	1½	51.4
soda	75	small slice: 75	8.0	2.3	3	56.3
white	66	large slice: 100	7.8	2.2	2	44.7
wholemeal	62	small slice: 64	8.8	2.7	2	41.8
Breadcrumbs, dried	101	15ml (1tbs): 10	11.6	1.9	15ml: 1½	77.5
Broccoli	5	140g(5oz): 25	3.1	Tr.	0	1.6
Brussels sprouts	5	115g (4oz): 20	2.8	Tr.	0	1.7
Butter	211	15g (½oz): 106	0.4	82.0	0	Tr.
Cabbage, red, raw	6	55g (2oz): 12	1.7	Tr.	0	3.5
Savoy, boiled	3	115g (4oz): 12	1.3	Tr.	0	1.1
white, raw	6	85g (3oz): 18	1.9	Tr.	0	3.8

FOOD OR DRINK	CALORIES per 25g (1oz)	CALORIES PER AVERAGE PORTION	PROTEIN PERCENTAGE	FAT PERCENTAGE	Cu PER 25g (1oz) unless portion stated	CARBOHYDRATE PERCENTAGE
Cakes					(slice)	
fancy, iced	116	average slice: 350	3.8	14.9	8	68.8
Madeira	112	average slice: 280	5.4	16.9	8¼	58.4
rich fruit	95	average slice: 285	3.7	11.0	10	58.3
rock	113	average piece: 240	5.4	16.3	7	60.2
sponge, fatless	86	average slice: 180	10.0	6.7	6	53.6
sponge, with fat	133	average slice: 278	6.4	26.5	6	53.2
Carrots, old, raw	6	about 12 each	0.7	Tr.	¼	5.4
boiled	5	115g (4oz): 20	0.6	Tr.	½	4.3
young, boiled	6	115g (4oz): 24	0.9	Tr.	¼	4.5
canned	5	115g (4oz): 20	0.7	Tr.	¼	4.4
Cauliflower	3	115g (4oz): 12	1.6	Tr.	0	0.8
Celeriac	4	85g (3oz): 12	1.6	Tr.	0	2.0
Celery, raw	2	about 4 each	0.9	Tr.	0	2.0
braised	1.5	85g (3oz): 4.5	0.6	Tr.	0	1.3
Cheese						
Camembert	86	55g (2oz): 172	22.8	23.2	0	Tr.
Cheddar	116	55g (2oz): 232	26.0	33.5	0	Tr.
cottage cheese	27	85g (3oz): 81	13.6	4.0	0	1.4
cream cheese	125	25g (1oz): 125	3.1	47.4	0	Tr.
curd cheese	47	55g (2oz): 94	16.9	9.9	0	1.8
Danish Blue	101	55g (2oz): 202	23.0	29.2	0	Tr.
Edam	88	55g (2oz): 176	24.4	22.9	0	Tr.
Parmesan	117	15ml (1tbs): 30	35.1	29.7	0	Tr.
processed cheese	89	25g (1oz): 89	21.5	25.0	0	Tr.
Stilton	115	55g (2oz): 230	25.6	40.0	0	Tr.
Cheesecake	120	average slice: 450	4.2	34.9	sl.: 4½	24.0
Cherries	13	115g (4oz): 52	0.6	Tr.	½	11.9
Chestnuts	49	55g (2oz): 98	2.0	2.7	2	36.6
Chicken, meat and skin	62	230g (8oz) grilled joint: 200	22.6	14.0	0	0
meat only, boiled	52	115g (4oz): 208	29.2	7.3	0	0
meat only, roast	42	115g (4oz): 168	24.8	5.4	0	0
Chicory, raw	3	55g (2oz): 6	0.8	Tr.	0	1.5
Chocolate, milk	151	55g (2oz): 302	8.4	30.3	3–4	59.4
plain	150	55g (2oz): 300	8.4	30.3	3–4	64.8
drinking	104	small cup: 215	5.5	6.0	5ml: ¾	77.4
Cider, dry	10	560ml (pint): 200	Tr.	0	10/ pint	2.6
sweet	12	560ml (pint): 350	Tr.	0	12½/pint	4.3
Coconut, fresh	100		3.2	36.0	0	3.7
desiccated	173	15ml (1tbs): 28	5.6	62.0	½	6.4
Cod, baked	27	140g (5oz): 135	21.4	1.2	0	0
fried in batter	57	170g (6oz): 342	19.6	10.3	½	7.5
grilled	27	170g (6oz): 162	20.8	1.3	0	0
steamed	24	170g (6oz): 144	18.6	0.9	0	0
Coffee, instant, black	28	cup: 0	14.6	0	0	11.0
roasted, black	82	cup: Tr.	10.4	15.4	0	28.5
Cola	11	185ml (6½fl oz): 80	Tr.	0	can: 4	10.5
Cornflakes	101	25g (1oz): 101	2.1	0.6	4¾	84.9
Cornflour	101	15ml (1tbs): 30	0.6	0.7	15 ml: 1	92.0
Crab, boiled	36	115g (4oz): 144	20.1	5.2	0	0
Cream, double	128	15ml (1tbs): 60	1.5	48.2	0	2.0
single	61	15ml (1tbs): 32	2.4	21.2	0	3.2
Cucumber	3	55g (2oz): 6	0.6	0.1	0	1.8
Currants	70	15ml (1tbs): 23	1.7	Tr.	3½	63.1
Currant buns	86	average bun: 150	7.4	7.6	5 ea.	54.5
Curry powder	67	15ml (1tbs): 14	9.5	10.8	15 ml: ¾	26.1
Custard, egg	34	170g (6oz): 204	5.8	6.0	½	11.0
made with powder	34	85g (3oz): 102	3.8	4.4	170 ml: 6	16.8
Damsons	11	115g (4oz): 44	0.5	Tr.	½	9.6
stewed with little sugar	20	115g (4oz): 80	0.3	Tr.	1	18.0
Dates, dried	71	about 35 each	2.0	Tr.	3½	63.9
Doughnuts	100	1 jam doughnut: 250	6.0	15.8	6 ea.	48.8
Dripping, beef	255		Tr.	99.0	0	0
Duck, roast, meat only	54	115g (4oz): 216	25.3	9.7	0	0
meat, fat and skin	97	115g (4oz): 388	19.6	29.0	0	0
Eclairs	107	average size: 200	4.1	24.0	4 ea.	38.2
Eel, stewed	57	115g (4oz): 228	20.6	13.2	0	0
Eggs, fresh or boiled	42	about 80 each	12.3	10.9	0	Tr.
fried	66	about 135 each				
omelette	54	plain, 3 eggs: 255				
poached	44	about 80 each				
scotch	80	about 300 each	11.6	20.9	½	11.8
whites	10		10.6	0.03	½	9.0
yolks	97		16.6	32.6	0	1.0

FOOD OR DRINK	CALORIES per 25g (1oz)	CALORIES PER AVERAGE PORTION	PROTEIN PERCENTAGE	FAT PERCENTAGE	Cu PER 25g (1oz) unless portion stated	CARBOHYDRATE PERCENTAGE
Endive	3		1.8	Tr.	0	1.0
Fat, low-fat spread	105	15g (½oz): 53	0	40.7	0	0
Fish fingers, fried	67	4, grilled: 200	13.5	12.7	1 ea.	17.2
Fish paste	48	15g (½oz): 24	15.3	10.4	¼–½	3.7
Frankfurters	78	about 215 each	9.5	25.0	½	3.0
French dressing	188	15ml (1tbs): 100	0.1	73.0	0	0.2
Fruit salad, canned	27	85g (3oz): 80	0.3	Tr.	1	25.0
Gelatin	97	15ml (1tsp): 22	84.4	Tr.	0	0
Gin (70% proof)	63	1 measure: 50	Tr.	0	3	Tr.
Gingerbread	107	average piece: 214	6.1	12.6	pce: 7	62.7
Golden Syrup	85	15ml (1tbs): 85	0.3	0	4½	79.0
Goose, roast meat	91	115g (4oz): 364	29.3	22.4	0	0
Gooseberries	5	115g (4oz): 20	1.1	Tr.	½	3.4
stewed with little sugar	14	115g (4oz): 56	0.9	Tr.	¾	12.5
Grapes, black	15	225g (½lb): 120	0.5	Tr.	¾	13.0
green	17	225g (½lb): 136	0.6	Tr.	1	15.3
Grapefruit	3	½ medium-sized: 15	0.3	Tr.	½:¾	2.5
canned	17	85g (3oz): 51	0.5	Tr.	1	15.5
juice, unsweetened	9	140ml (5fl oz): 45	0.3	Tr.	½	7.9
Greengages	13	115g (4oz): 52	0.8	Tr.	¾	11.8
Ground ginger	74		7.4	3.3	3½	60.0
Grouse, roast	49	115g (4oz): 200	30.1	5.3	0	0
Guinea fowl, roast	60	115g (4oz): 240	32.5	8.2	0	0
Haddock, steamed	21	140g (5oz): 105	17.3	0.6	0	0
fried (with bones)	46	140g (5oz): 230	19.7	7.6	0	3.3
smoked and steamed	19	140g (5oz): 95	15.1	0.6	0	0
Haggis, boiled	89	115g (4oz): 356	10.7	21.7	1	19.2
Halibut, steamed	37	140g (5oz): 185	23.8	4.0	0	0
Ham, canned	34	115g (4oz): 136	18.4	5.1	0	0
and pork, chopped	77	55g (2oz): 154	14.4	23.6	0	0
Hare, stewed	40	140g (5oz): 200	21.8	5.8	0	0
Heart, ox, stewed	51	115g (4oz): 204	31.4	5.9	0	0
sheep, roast	68	115g (4oz): 272	26.1	14.7	0	0
Herring, fried	59	140g (5oz): 295	20.3	13.3	0	1.3
grilled	39	140g (5oz): 195	13.9	8.8	0	0
Honey	82	5ml (1tsp): 20	0.4	Tr.	5 ml: 1	76.4
Ice cream, dairy	48	115ml (4fl oz): 96	3.7	6.6	1½	24.8
non-dairy	47	115ml (4fl oz): 94	3.3	8.2	1	20.7
Jam	74	5ml (1 tsp): 17	0.6	0	4	69.0
Jelly	17	55g (2oz): 34	1.4	0	¾	14.2
Kidneys, lamb's, fried	44	115g (4oz): 176	24.6	6.3	0	0
ox, stewed	49	115g (4oz): 196	25.6	7.7	0	0
pig, stewed	44	115g (4oz): 176	24.4	6.1	0	0
Kippers, baked	59	115g (4oz): 236	25.5	11.4	0	0
with bones, grilled	32	170g (6oz): 192	13.8	6.2	0	0
Lamb						
breast, roast	117	140g (5oz): 585	19.1	37.1	0	0
cutlets, grilled	106	140g (5oz): 530	23.0	30.9	0	0
leg, roast	76	115g (4oz): 304	26.1	17.9	0	0
loin chops, well grilled	101	average chop: 200	23.5	29.0	0	0
scrag and neck, stewed	83	140g (5oz): 415	25.6	21.1	0	0
shoulder, roast	90	115g (4oz): 360	19.9	26.3	0	0
Leeks	7	115g (4oz): 28	1.8	Tr.	½ ea.	4.6
Lemon, whole	4	15ml (1tbs) juice: 1	0.8	Tr.	1 ea.	3.2
Lemon curd	81	5ml (1tsp): 12	0.6	5.1	3½	62.7
Lemon sole, fried with bones	49	140g (5oz): 245	12.7	10.3	½	7.4
steamed	18	140g (5oz): 90	14.6	0.6	0	0
Lemonade	6	140ml (5fl oz): 54	Tr.	0	¼	5.6
Lentils, boiled	28	55g (2oz): 56	7.6	0.5	1	17.0
Lettuce	3		1.0	0.4	0	1.2
Lime juice cordial (undiluted)	32	average glass: 15	0.1	0	1½	29.8
Liver, calf's, fried	73	115g (4oz): 292	26.9	13.2	0	7.3
chicken, fried	55	115g (4oz): 220	20.7	10.9	0	3.4
lamb's, fried	66	115g (4oz): 264	22.9	14.0	0	3.9
ox, stewed	57	115g (4oz): 228	24.8	9.5	0	3.6
pig's, stewed	54	115g (4oz): 216	25.6	8.1	0	3.6
sausage	89	55g (2oz): 178	12.9	26.9	0	4.3
Lobster, boiled, meat only	34	115g (4oz): 136	22.1	3.4	0	0
Loganberries	5	115g (4oz): 20	1.1	Tr.	¼	3.4
Luncheon meat	89	55g (2oz): 178	12.6	26.9	¼	5.5

FOOD OR DRINK	CALORIES per 25g (1oz)	CALORIES PER AVERAGE PORTION	PROTEIN PERCENTAGE	FAT PERCENTAGE	Cu PER 25g (1oz) unless portion stated	CARBOHYDRATE PERCENTAGE
Lychees, canned	19	85g (3oz): 57	0.4	Tr.	1	17.7
Macaroni, boiled	33	55g (2oz): 66	4.3	0.6	1½	25.2
Mackerel, with bones, fried	39	170g (6oz): 234	15.7	8.3	0	0
Mandarins, canned	16	115g ((4oz): 64	0.6	Tr.	1	14.2
Mango, fresh	17	about 60 each	0.5	Tr.	1	15.3
canned	22	115g (4oz): 88	0.3	Tr.	1	20.3
Margarine	209	15g (½oz): 105	0.1	81.0	0	0.1
Marmalade	74	5ml (1tsp): 17	0.1	0	4	69.5
Marrow	2	115g (4oz): 8	0.4	Tr.	0	1.4
Marzipan	126		8.7	24.9	3	49.2
Mayonnaise	205	15ml (1tbs): 96	1.8	78.9	0	0.1
low calorie	101	15ml (1tbs): 47	3.2	35.8	¼	4.7
Melon						
cantaloupe	4	average slice: 24	0.6	Tr.	0	3.3
honeydew	4	average slice: 24	0.4	Tr.	0	3.1
watermelon	3	average slice: 18	0.2	Tr.	0	2.7
Meringues	109	1 fresh cream: 150	5.3	0	7 ea.	95.6
Milk						
condensed, sweetened	92	15ml (1tbs): 50	8.3	9.0	3	55.5
goat's	20	560ml (pint): 400	3.3	4.5	pt.: 5	4.6
skimmed, dried	101	560ml (pint): 200	36.4	1.3	pt.: 5½	52.8
skimmed, fresh	9	560ml (pint): 200	3.4	0.1	pt.: 5½	5.0
whole fresh	19	560ml (pint): 370	3.3	3.8	pt.: 5	5.10
Mincemeat	67	15ml (1tbs): 42	0.6	4.3	15 ml: 2	62.1
Muesli	105	55g (2oz): 210	12.9	7.5	4	66.2
Mussels, boiled	25	115g (4oz): 100	17.2	2.0	0	Tr.
Mushrooms	4	85g (3oz): 12	1.8	0.6	0	0
fried	60	85g (3oz): 180	2.2	22.3	0	0
Mustard and cress	3		1.6	Tr.	0	0.9
Nectarines	13	about 25 each	0.9	Tr.	¾	11.4
Oatmeal, raw	115	15ml (1tbs): 37	12.4	8.7	4	72.8
porridge	13	115g (4oz): 52	1.4	0.9	½	8.2
Okra	5	115g (4oz): 20	2.0	Tr.	0	2.3
Olive oil	257	15ml (1tbs): 123	Tr.	99.9	0	0
Onions	7	55g (2oz): 14	0.9	Tr.	¼	5.2
boiled	4	85g (3oz): 12	0.6	2.7	0	2.7
fried	99	55g (2oz): 198	1.8	33.3	½	10.1
spring	10		0.9	8.5	½	8.5
Oranges	10	about 40 each	0.8	Tr.	2 ea.	8.5
juice, canned	9	115ml (4fl oz): 36	0.4	Tr.	½	8.5
juice, fresh	11	115ml (4fl oz): 44	0.6	Tr.	½	9.4
Oxtail, stewed with bones	26	200g (7oz): 182	11.6	5.1	0	0
Oysters, without shells, raw	15	about 5 each	10.8	0.9	0	Tr.
Pancakes (dessert)	88	about 130 each	6.1	16.3	5 ea.	36.2
Parsley	6		5.2	Tr.	0	Tr.
Parsnips	16	115g (4oz): 64	1.3	Tr.	¾	13.5
Partridge, roast, on bone	36	200g (7oz): 252	22.0	4.3	0	0
Pastry, flaky	161		5.8	40.5	3	47.4
short	151		7.7	33.4	3	54.9
Peaches	9	about 40 each	0.6	Tr.	½	7.9
canned	25	115g (4oz): 100	0.4	Tr.	1¼	22.9
Peanuts	163	55g (2oz): 326	24.3	49.0	½	8.6
Peanut butter	178		22.6	53.7	¾	13.1
Pears	8	about 32 each	0.2	Tr.	½	7.6
canned	22	115g (4oz): 88	0.4	Tr.	1	20.0
Peas, raw	19		5.8	0.4	½	10.6
boiled	15	15ml (1tbs): 15	5.0	0.4	½	7.7
chick peas	41	55g (2oz): 82	8.0	3.3	1¼	22.0
dried, boiled	29	15ml (1tbs): 30	6.9	0.4	1	19.1
frozen, boiled	12	55g (2oz): 24	5.4	0.4	¼	4.3
processed	23	55g (2oz): 46	6.2	0.4	¾	13.7
split, boiled	34	15ml (1tbs): 35	8.3	0.3	1¼	21.9
Peppers	4	55g (2oz): 8	0.9	0.4	¼	2.2
boiled	4	140g (5oz): 20	0.9	0.4	0	1.8
Pheasant, roast, on bone	38	170g (6oz): 228	20.3	5.9	0	0
Pies						
Fruit (individual)	105	about 360 each	4.3	15.5	9 ea.	56.7
lemon meringue	92	average slice: 368	4.5	14.6	sl.: 4	46.4
mince	124	about 135 each	4.3	20.7	5¼ ea.	61.7
Pigeon, roast, on bone	29	250g (9oz) bird: 260	12.2	5.8	0	0
Pilchards, canned	36	55g (2oz): 72	18.8	5.4	0	0.7
Pineapple	13	115g (4oz): 52	0.5	Tr.	¾	11.6
canned	22	1 drained ring: 35	0.3	Tr.	1	20.2

FOOD OR DRINK	CALORIES per 25g (1oz)	CALORIES PER AVERAGE PORTION	PROTEIN PERCENTAGE	FAT PERCENTAGE	Cu PER 25g (1oz) unless portion stated	CARBOHYDRATE PERCENTAGE
juice	15	140ml (5fl oz): 75	0.4	0.1		13.4
Plaice, fried in batter	80	140g (5oz): 400	15.8	18.0	¾	14.4
fried in breadcrumbs	65	140g (5oz): 325	18.0	13.7	½	8.6
steamed fillet	27	140g (5oz): 135	18.9	1.9	0	0
steamed whole	14	140g (5oz): 70	10.2	1.0	0	0
Plums	10	about 15 each	0.5	Tr.	½	9.0
stewed with little sugar	17	115g (4oz): 68	0.4	Tr.	1	15.3
Pork						
belly rashers, grilled	114	85g (3oz): 342	21.1	34.8	0	0
loin chops, well grilled	95	average chop: 200	28.5	24.2	0	0
leg, roast	82	115g (4oz): 328	26.9	19.8	0	0
pie, individual	107	about 320 each	9.8	27.0	4½ ea.	24.9
Port	45	55ml (2fl oz): 90	0.1	0	¾	12.0
Potatoes						
baked with skin	24	200g (7oz): 168	2.1	0.1	1	20.3
boiled, new	22	140g (5oz): 110	1.6	0.1	1	18.3
boiled, old	23	140g (5oz): 115	1.4	0.1	1	19.7
chips	72	140g (5oz): 360	3.8	10.9	140g: 10	37.3
crisps	152	small packet: 102	6.3	35.9	2¾	49.3
instant powder, made up	20	40ml (2 heaped tbs): 105	2.0	0.2	1	16.1
mashed	34	140g (5oz): 170	1.5	5.0	1	18.0
roast	45	140g (5oz): 225	2.8	4.8	1½	27.3
Prawns, boiled and peeled	31	55g (2oz): 62	22.6	1.8	0	0
Prunes, dried and stewed	21	115g (4oz): 82	1.1	Tr.	1	18.6
Puddings						
bread and butter	45	140g (5oz): 225	6.1	7.8	½	17.2
Christmas	87	170g (6oz): 522	5.2	11.6	2¾	47.6
milk	37	115g (4oz): 148	4.1	4.2	1	20.4
Quiche	112	average slice: 560	14.7	28.1	sl.: 5	21.1
Rabbit, stewed with bone	26	200g (7oz): 182	13.9	3.9	0	0
Radishes	4	15g (½oz): 2	1.0	Tr.	0	2.8
Raisins	70	15ml (1tbs): 26	1.1	Tr.	3½	64.4
Raspberries	7	85g (3oz): 21	0.9	Tr.	¼	5.6
canned	25	115g (4oz): 100	0	Tr.	1	20.0
Rhubarb, stewed without sugar	1½	115g (4oz): 6	0.6	Tr.	0	0.9
stewed with little sugar	13	115g (4oz): 52	0.5	Tr.	½	11.4
Rice, boiled	35	140g (5oz): 175	2.2	0.3	1½	29.6
Salad cream	89	15ml (1tbs): 42	1.9	27.4	¾	15.3
Salad dressing, low calorie	37	15ml (1tbs): 17	1.6	8.7	½	12.3
Salami	140	55g (2oz): 280	19.3	45.2	0	1.9
Salmon, steamed	56	140g (5oz): 280	20.1	13.0	0	0
canned	44	55g (2oz): 88	20.3	8.2	0	0
smoked	41	55g (2oz): 82	25.4	4.5	0	0
Sardines, in oil, drained	62	1 fish: 60	23.7	13.6	0	0
in tomato	51	1 fish: 50	17.8	11.6	0	0
Sausage roll, flaky pastry	137	55g (2oz) roll: 274	7.2	36.2	55g: 3¾	33.1
Sausages						
beef, fried	77	1 large: 110	12.9	18.0	½ ea.	14.9
grilled	76	1 large: 110	13.0	17.3	½ ea.	15.2
pork, fried	91	1 large: 120	13.8	24.5	½ ea.	11.0
grilled	91	1 large: 120	13.3	24.6	½ ea.	11.5
Scallops, steamed	30	115g (4oz): 120	23.2	1.4	0	Tr.
Scampi, fried	90	140g (5oz): 450	12.2	17.6	1½	28.9
Seakale	2	115g (4oz): 8	1.4	Tr.	0	0.6
Semolina	100	15ml (1tbs): 35	10.7	1.8	4¼	77.5
Sherry, dry	33	55ml (2fl oz): 66	0.2	0	55 ml: 2	1.4
medium	34	55ml (2fl oz): 68	0.1	0	55 ml: 3	3.6
sweet	39	55ml (2fl oz): 78	0.3	0	55 ml: 4	6.9
Shrimps, boiled	33	55g (2oz): 66	23.8	2.4	0	0
Skate, fried in batter	57	170g (6oz): 342	17.9	12.1	¼	4.9
Sole, steamed	24	170g (6oz): 144	17.6	1.3	0	0
fried	78	170g (6oz): 468	20.1	18.4	0	0
Soup						
canned bone and vegetable broth	16	bowl: 56	3.7	4.6	0	1.1
canned chicken noodle	6	bowl: 20	0.8	0.3	bowl: 1	3.7
canned cream of chicken	16	bowl: 56	1.7	3.8	bowl: 1½	4.5
canned cream of tomato	15	bowl: 53	0.8	20.9	bowl: 2	11.8
canned lentil	26	bowl: 93	4.4	3.7	bowl: 2	11.9
Spaghetti, boiled	33	55g (2oz): 66	4.2	0.3	1½	26.0
Spinach	9	115g (4oz): 36	5.1	0.5	0	1.4
Sprats, fried with bones	111	115g (4oz): 444	21.9	33.4	0	0
Spring greens	3	115g (4oz): 12	1.7	Tr.	0	0.9
Strawberries, fresh	7	85g (3oz): 21	0.6	Tr.	¼	6.2

FOOD OR DRINK	CALORIES per 25g (1oz)	CALORIES PER AVERAGE PORTION	PROTEIN PERCENTAGE	FAT PERCENTAGE	Cu PER 25g (1oz) unless portion stated	CARBOHYDRATE PERCENTAGE
Suet, shredded	236	15ml (1tbs): 77	Tr.	86.7	¾	12.1
Sugar, demerara	113	5ml (1tsp): 14	0.5	O	tsp: 1	99.5
white	113	5ml (1tsp): 14	Tr.	O	tsp: 1	99.5
Sultanas	71	15ml (1tbs): 25	1.8	Tr.	3¾	64.7
Swedes	5	115g (4oz): 20	0.9	Tr.	2 tbs: ½	3.8
Sweetbreads, lamb, fried	66	115g (4oz): 264	19.4	14.6	O	5.6
Sweetcorn	35	large cob: 85	4.1	2.3	1¼	22.8
canned kernels	22	15ml (1tbs): 12	2.9	0.5	1¼	22.8
Sweet potatoes	24	4:96	1.1	0.6	1	20.1
Sweets						
boiled	93		Tr.	Tr.	5	87.3
peppermints	112		0.5	O	5¾	102.2
toffee	123		2.1	17.2	4	71.1
Tangerine	10	about 30 each	0.9	Tr.	1 ea.	8.0
Tarts						
custard, individual	82	about 225 each	5.9	16.9	5 ea.	29.6
jam, individual	110	about 115 each	3.5	14.9	4½ ea.	62.8
treacle	106	average slice: 318	3.8	14.0	sl.: 5	61.3
Tea, with milk		cup: 20	19.6	2.0	O	3.0
Tomatoes, raw	4	average tomato: 8	0.9	Tr.	O	2.8
fried	20	average tomato: 20	1.0	5.9	O	3.3
canned	3	200g (7oz) can: 21	1.1	Tr.	O	2.0
juice	4	140ml (5fl oz): 20	0.7	Tr.	¼	3.4
ketchup	28	15ml (1tbs): 16	2.1	Tr.	1¼	24.0
purée	19	15ml (1tbs): 18	6.1	Tr.	¾	11.4
Tongue, sheep, boiled	83	55g (2oz): 166	18.2	24.0	O	O
ox, boiled	84	55g (2oz): 168	19.5	23.9	O	O
Treacle	73	15m (1tbs): 45	1.2	O	4	67.2
Trifle	46	140g (5oz): 230	3.5	6.1	140g: 6½	24.3
Tripe, stewed	29	140g (5oz): 145	14.8	4.5	O	Tr.
Trout, steamed	25	200g (7oz): 175	15.5	3.0	O	O
Tuna, in oil, drained	60	85g (3oz): 180	29.0	8.0	O	O
Turkey, meat and skin	49	140g (5oz): 245	28.0	6.5	O	O

FOOD OR DRINK	CALORIES per 25g (1oz)	CALORIES PER AVERAGE PORTION	PROTEIN PERCENTAGE	FAT PERCENTAGE	Cu PER 25g (1oz) unless portion stated	CARBOHYDRATE PERCENTAGE
meat only, roast	40	140g (5oz): 200	28.8	2.7	O	O
Turnips	4	115g (4oz): 16	0.7	0.3	115g: ½	2.3
Veal, cutlet, fried	61	115g (4oz): 244	31.4	8.1	¼	4.4
fillet, roast	66	115g (4oz): 264	31.6	11.5	O	O
jellied	36	55g (2oz): 72	25.0	2.8	O	O
Vegetable oil	257	15ml (1tbs): 76	Tr.	99.9	O	O
Venison, roast	57	115g (4oz): 228	35.0	6.4	O	O
Vermouth, dry	34	55ml (2fl oz): 68	0.1	O	55 ml: 4	5.5
sweet	43	55ml (2fl oz): 86	Tr.	O	55 ml: 4	15.9
Vodka (70% proof)	63	1 measure: 50	Tr.	O	3	Tr.
Walnuts	150	Walnut half: 15	10.6	51.5	¼	5.0
Watercress	4		2.9	Tr.	O	0.7
Whelks, boiled	26	115g (4oz): 104	18.5	1.9	O	Tr.
Whisky (70% proof)	63	1 measure: 50	Tr.	O	3	Tr.
Whitebait, fried	150	115g (4oz): 600	19.5	47.5	¼	5.3
Whiting, fillet, steamed	26	140g (5oz): 130	14.3	0.6	O	O
fillet, fried	54	140g (5oz): 270	16.3	9.3	¼	6.3
on bone, steamed	18	200g (7oz): 126	14.3	0.6	O	O
on bone, fried	49	200g (7oz): 343	16.3	9.3	¼	6.3
Wine, white, dry	19	115ml (4fl oz): 76	0.1	O	115 ml: 4	0.6
medium	21	115ml (4fl oz): 84	0.1	O	115 ml: 4	3.4
sweet	27	115ml (4fl oz): 108	0.2	O	115 ml: 5	5.9
sparkling	22	115ml (4fl oz): 88	0.3	O	115ml: 4½	1.4
red	19	115ml (4fl oz): 76	0.2	O	115 ml: 4	0.3
Winkles, boiled	21	55g (2oz): 42	15.3	1.4	O	Tr.
Yam	34	115g (4oz): 136	1.6	0.1	1½	29.8
Yoghurt, natural	15	140g (5oz) carton: 75	3.0	1.0	car.: 3	6.2
fruit	27	140g (5oz) carton: 135–145	4.3	0.7	car.: 4½–5	16.2
Yorkshire pudding	61	115g (4oz): 244	6.8	10.1	1½	25.8

Index

ACKNOWLEDGMENTS

Photography:
Chris Holland
Paul Kemp (pages 14–35)

Make-up: Mary Lou

Hair: Ann Mathews at Toni and Guy

Stylist: Bonnie Estridge

The photograph on page 70 is reproduced by permission of Alastair Black.

The publishers would also like to thank the following for providing materials and equipment used in photography: Adidas, Laura Ashley, Boots, Braun, Condor Cycles, The Dance Centre, Harrods, Inside Out Shop, Marks and Spencer, MFI Furniture, Natural Shoe Store.

Thanks are also due to Iris Marsaglia and the West Side Health Club for advising on the exercises for photography, and to the British Nutrition Foundation for their help and advice. The figures in the table on pages 76–79 are based on data compiled from *Composition of Foods* (HMSO).